OMAD DIET 2025

110 Recipes A New Approach to Wellbeing and Weight Loss Revolutionize Your Life with Just One Meal a Day

KLARLOCK

DISCLAIMER

This book aims to provide useful and informative material on the topics covered in the publication. It is sold with the understanding that the author and publisher are not engaged in rendering any personal medical, health care, or other professional services in the book. The reader should consult his or her physician, health care provider, or other competent professional before adopting any suggestions in this book or drawing any conclusions. The author and publisher expressly disclaim any responsibility for any liability, loss, or risk, personal or otherwise, arising, directly or indirectly, from the use and application of any contents of this book.

NOTE

All the recipes in this book are designed for four people. For this quantity, the ingredients indicated in the recipes must be considered. If you need to change the portion, it is recommended to proportionally adjust the doses of the ingredients. It is also recommended to carefully follow the preparation and cooking instructions to obtain the best result. In the context of this book, when we refer to "a cup" as a unit of measurement for ingredients, we mean using a standard kitchen cup with a capacity of approximately 240 milliliters. It is essential to use a measuring cup to get the right quantities of ingredients. If you don't have a measuring cup, you can use a graduated measuring cup, making sure to correctly correspond to the proportions indicated. Here are some examples 1 Cup of flour 100 gr. 1 cup of rice 200 gr. 1 Cup of Quinoa 200 gr

TABLE OF CONTENT

RECIPES FIRST DISHES

RECIPES SECOND DISHES

SIDE DISH RECIPES

INTRODUCTION TO THE OMAD DIET

WHAT IS THE OMAD DIET

HISTORY AND ORIGINS OF THE OMAD DIET

The OMAD Diet, an acronym for "One Meal A Day", is a form of intermittent fasting that involves consuming all your daily calories in a single eating session. This diet is based on the idea of reducing the frequency of meals to improve health and facilitate weight loss. What is the OMAD Diet The OMAD Diet is a dietary practice that involves consuming just one complete meal a day, generally in a one-hour window, while fasting for the remaining 23 hours. This diet is one of the most extreme variations of intermittent fasting, which includes other forms such as 16:8 (16 hours of fasting and 8 hours of eating) and 5:2 (five days of normal diet and two days of calorie restriction). History and Origins of the OMAD Diet The concept of eating a single meal a day is not new. Different cultures and religious traditions have practiced fasting for centuries as part of their spiritual and health routines. However, the OMAD Diet has gained popularity in recent years thanks to anecdotal reports of people experiencing notable benefits in terms of weight loss and overall well-being. Its simplicity and potential to improve metabolic health have attracted the attention of those seeking effective weight management and health solutions. Potential Benefits Numerous studies suggest that intermittent fasting may offer a number of health benefits, and the OMAD Diet is no exception. Potential benefits include: Weight Loss: By reducing the number of meals you eat, many people find it easier to maintain a calorie deficit, which is essential for weight loss. Improvement of

Metabolism: Fasting can increase insulin sensitivity and promote the production of hormones that help burn fat. **Simplicity and Convenience:** Eating once a day can simplify meal planning and reduce the time spent preparing food. **Mental Benefits:** Some practitioners report increased mental clarity and focus during fasting periods. **Longevity and Cellular Health:** Animal studies suggest that fasting may promote longevity and improve cellular health, although further research is needed to confirm these effects in humans. The OMAD Diet represents a significant challenge and is not suitable for everyone. It is important to carefully consider your nutritional needs and consult a doctor or nutritionist before embarking on this diet.

BASIC PRINCIPLES OF THE OMAD DIET

The OMAD (One Meal A Day) Diet is based on a simple but challenging concept: consuming all your daily calories in a single meal. This approach to intermittent fasting offers potential benefits for weight loss, metabolic health, and overall well-being, but requires a clear understanding of its basic principles to be practiced effectively and safely. How the OMAD Diet Works The OMAD Diet involves eating just one full meal a day, generally within a one-hour window. During the remaining 23 hours, you fast. This approach can be flexible with meal timing, depending on personal preferences and daily commitments, but it is important to maintain the fasting window to achieve maximum benefits. Eating Window and Fasting 1. Eating Window The eating window is the period during which you eat your daily meal.

It can vary, but usually lasts an hour. During this time, it is essential to consume a nutritious, balanced meal that provides all the calories and nutrients needed to sustain the body until the next meal. 2. Fasting Period: During the 23 hours of fasting, it is recommended to consume only water, tea, black coffee and other calorie-free drinks. Avoiding any caloric food or drink is crucial to maintaining the fasting state and allowing the body to benefit from the metabolic processes that are activated during this period. Choosing Foods Choosing the right foods is essential to the success of the OMAD Diet. A single meal a day should be sufficient to meet your daily nutritional needs, so it is important to include a variety of nutritious foods: Protein: Lean meat, fish, eggs, legumes and tofu are excellent sources of protein essential for the repair and maintenance of body tissues. Complex Carbohydrates: Whole grains, starchy vegetables and legumes they provide long-lasting energy and fiber for digestion. Healthy Fats: Avocados, nuts, seeds, olive oil and fatty fish like salmon are rich in essential fatty acids that support heart and brain health. Vegetables: A wide range of vegetables, especially leafy greens, provide vitamins, minerals and antioxidants crucial for overall well-being. Fruit: Fresh fruit is a natural source of vitamins, minerals and fibre, but it is important not to overdo it due to the natural sugar content. Caloric and Nutritional Balance It is essential that the single meal consumed in the OMAD Diet is well balanced from a caloric and nutritional point of view. Be sure to include an adequate combination of macronutrients (proteins, carbohydrates and fats) and micronutrients (vitamins and minerals) to support all body functions and prevent nutritional deficiencies. Personalization and Listening to the Body The OMAD Diet can be personalized according to needs individual. It's important to listen to your body and adapt your approach as needed. Some people may start with a larger eating window and gradually reduce it, while others may find the one-hour format comfortable right away. Awareness and Mindfulness Practicing mindfulness during a meal can improve the OMAD Diet experience. Eating slowly, savoring each bite and listening to your satiety cues can help ensure your meal is satisfying and nutritious. By following these basic principles, you can adopt the OMAD Diet safely and effectively, enjoying the potential benefits to your overall health and well-being.

HOW TO GET STARTED WITH THE OMAD DIET

The OMAD (One Meal A Day) Diet may seem challenging, but with proper preparation and a gradual transition, it can become a sustainable and beneficial regimen. Here is a detailed guide on how to get started with the OMAD Diet. Mental and Physical Preparation 1. Educate yourself: Before you begin, it is essential to fully understand how the OMAD Diet works and what its benefits and potential risks are. Reading articles, scientific studies and testimonials can provide a solid foundation of knowledge. 2. Consult a Professional: Talking to a doctor or nutritionist is important, especially if you have pre-existing medical conditions. A professional can help determine if the OMAD Diet is right and how to adapt it to your personal needs. 3. Mental Preparation: The OMAD Diet requires discipline and willpower. Prepare mentally for fasting periods and develop strategies to manage hunger can make a big difference. Gradual Transition 1. Start with Intermittent Fasting: Before switching to just one meal a day, starting with a less rigorous intermittent fasting regimen, such as 16:8 (16 hours fasting and 8 hours eating), can help the body to adapt gradually. 2. Gradually Reduce Meals: Slowly reduce the number of meals per day. Going from three meals a day to two, and finally to just one, allows the body to adapt without shock. 3. Monitor Your Body's Reactions: During the transition, it is important to listen to your body and monitor how it reacts. Make adjustments if you experience excessive hunger, fatigue or other negative symptoms. Meal Planning 1. Choice of Meal Time: Decide the meal time based on your personal commitments and energy needs. Some people prefer to eat for lunch, others for dinner. Consistency is important to establish a routine. 2. Nutritious and Balanced Meal: Make sure that the single meal is nutritious and balanced.

Include a combination of proteins, complex carbohydrates, healthy fats, vegetables and fruits to meet nutritional needs. 3. Meal Preparation: Planning and preparing meals in advance can help ensure they are balanced and nutritious. This also reduces stress and the temptation to opt for less healthy food choices. ### Tips for Success 1. Hydration: Drinking plenty of water during the fasting period is key. Water helps you stay hydrated and can help control hunger. Sugar-free tea and coffee are also permitted. 2. Hunger Management: Distracting yourself with activities such as reading, work, exercise or hobbies can help manage hunger during fasting. 3. Exercise: Regular physical activity can support weight loss and improve overall well-being. It is important to listen to your body and adapt the intensity of the exercise according to your energy. 4. Sleep: Getting enough sleep is important.

Good sleep supports metabolism, mental and physical health. Monitoring and Adaptation 1. Keep a Food Diary: Recording what you eat, how you feel and any changes in your weight and health can help you identify what works best and what may need to be changed. 2. Flexible Adjustments: Be open to making adjustments if necessary. If one meal a day is too difficult, consider a slightly longer eating window and gradually reduce it. 3. Regular Checkups: Have regular checkups with a doctor to monitor your health and make sure the OMAD Diet is not causing any adverse effects. Getting started with the OMAD Diet requires commitment and preparation, but with a gradual transition and proper planning, you can adopt this diet effectively and sustainably.

BENEFITS OF THE OMAD DIET

The OMAD (One Meal A Day) Diet has gained popularity due to the numerous benefits that many practitioners report. This intermittent fasting regimen, characterized by eating just one meal a day, can offer significant benefits for weight loss, metabolic health, and overall well-being. Weight Loss One of the most immediate and visible benefits of the OMAD Diet is weight loss. Here's how this regimen can help: Reduce Calorie Intake: Eating just one meal a day often leads to a lower total calorie burn, helping to create a calorie deficit essential for weight loss. Increased Metabolism: Some studies suggest that intermittent fasting may increase insulin sensitivity and improve metabolism, making it easier to use fat as an energy source. Control Hunger and Cravings: Focusing on just one meal can help reduce cravings and improve control appetite, making it easier to avoid snacking and unhealthy food. Improved Metabolism The OMAD Diet can have positive effects on metabolism and overall metabolic health: Insulin Sensitivity: Prolonged fasting can improve insulin sensitivity, reducing the risk of developing type 2 diabetes. Hormone Regulation: Fasting can positively influence the production of hormones such as leptin and ghrelin, which regulate hunger and satiety. Increased HGH Production: Intermittent fasting can increase the production of human growth hormone (HGH), which supports fat loss and muscle growth. Mental Health Benefits In addition to the physical benefits, the OMAD Diet can also positively affect mental health: Improved Concentration and Mental Clarity: Many practitioners report feeling more focused and mentally clear during periods of fasting. Stress Reduction: Simplifying your eating routine, can reduce stress related to meal planning and food decisions. Increased Discipline and Control: Following a strict fasting regime can increase your sense of discipline and personal control. Other Health Benefits The OMAD Diet may offer additional overall health benefits:

Cardiovascular Health: Intermittent fasting may improve markers of cardiovascular health, such as cholesterol levels and blood pressure. Reduced Inflammation: Some studies suggest that fasting can reduce inflammation in the body, decreasing the risk of chronic disease. Improved Digestive Health: Reducing meal frequency can give your digestive system a break, improving digestion and gut health. Longevity and Cellular Health There is preliminary evidence to suggest that the OMAD Diet may positively influence longevity and cellular health: Autophagy: Prolonged fasting can activate the process of autophagy, in which cells eliminate debris and damaged components, promoting regeneration mobile phone. The OMAD Diet has many potential benefits, but it is important to practice it consciously and under the guidance of a health professional, especially for individuals with pre-existing medical conditions.

CONCLUSION AND FUTURE OF THE OMAD DIET

Conclusion The OMAD (One Meal A Day) diet has gained popularity as a diet that promises significant benefits for health and weight management. Numerous studies have highlighted the potential benefits of this approach, including: Weight Loss: Daily calorie restriction and eating just one meal a day can aid in weight loss and reduction of fat mass Improved Metabolic Health: The OMAD diet can improve metabolic flexibility and insulin sensitivity, contributing to the prevention and management of type 2 diabetes Liver Health: Reduction of fatty liver index thanks to the decrease in total caloric intake Composition of the Intestinal Microbiota: Effects positive on the composition of the intestinal microbiota, with beneficial implications for overall metabolic health, Future of the Diet

OMAD The future of the OMAD diet appears promising, but requires further research to consolidate existing evidence and explore new areas of interest. Here are some crucial aspects that could define the future of the OMAD diet: 1. Continued Research: Further large-scale clinical studies are needed to confirm the long-term benefits of the OMAD diet and to better understand its effects on different populations and health conditions . 2. Personalization: The development of personalized approaches to the OMAD diet, based on individual factors such as age, gender, level of physical activity and pre-existing health conditions, could improve its effectiveness and adherence. 3. Technology Integration: The use of advanced technologies such as health tracking apps, wearable devices and artificial intelligence algorithms could support people following the OMAD diet, offering real-time feedback and personalized advice. 4. Education and Awareness: Increase the

Awareness and education regarding the benefits and risks of the OMAD diet can help people make informed decisions. Educational programs and online resources could play a key role in this process. 5. Integration with Other Diets: Studying how the OMAD diet can be combined with other nutritional approaches, such as plant-based or ketogenic diets, could provide new options for improving health and well-being. In conclusion, while the OMAD diet has been shown to offer several health benefits, its success depends on customization and long-term adherence. With continued research and technological innovation, the OMAD diet could become an increasingly integrated and supported component of the healthy diets of the future.

RECIPES APPETIZERS

TOMATO BRUSCHETTE

Preparation time: 10 minutes

Cooking time: 5 minutes

Doses: 1 person

Ingredients:

2 slices of homemade bread

1 ripe tomato

1 clove of garlic

2 tablespoons of oil

extra virgin olive oil

Fresh basil to taste

Salt and Pepper To Taste

Preparation:

Wash the tomato and cut it into cubes. Finely chop the garlic and basil. In a large bowl, mix the diced tomatoes, minced garlic, basil, extra virgin olive oil, salt and pepper. Toast the slices of homemade bread on the grill or in the oven until golden brown. Rub each slice of toasted bread with a clove of garlic. Spread the tomato and basil mixture over the bread slices. Serve immediately and enjoy.

Nutritional values (per serving):

Calories: 125 kcal

Fat: 6 g

Carbohydrates: 15 g

Protein: 4 g

Fibers: 2 g

CAPRESE WITH BUFFALO MOZZARELLA

Preparation time: 5 minutes

Cooking time: 0 minutes

Doses: 1 person

Ingredients:

100 g of fresh buffalo mozzarella

1 ripe tomato

Fresh basil to taste

Extra virgin olive oil to taste

Salt and Pepper To Taste

Preparation:

Wash the tomato and cut it into slices about 1 cm thick. Cut the buffalo mozzarella into slices slightly thicker than the tomatoes. Arrange the tomatoes and mozzarella in layers on a serving plate, alternating them. Garnish with fresh basil leaves. Drizzle with a drizzle of extra virgin olive oil. Salt and pepper to taste. Serve immediately and enjoy.

Nutritional values (per serving):

Calories: 200 kcal

Fat: 15 g

Carbohydrates: 7 g

Protein: 12 g

Fibres: 1 g

CROSTINI WITH LIVER PATÉ

Preparation time: 15 minutes

Cooking time: 20 minutes

Doses: 1 person

Ingredients:

For the liver pâté:

100 g of chicken livers

1/4 medium onion

1/4 carrot

1/4 stalk of celery

1 tablespoon extra virgin olive oil

1 tablespoon butter

1/4 glass of dry white wine

1 anchovy in oil

1 tablespoon capers

1 sprig of sage

1 sprig of rosemary

Salt and Pepper To Taste

For the croutons:

2 slices of homemade bread

1 tablespoon extra virgin olive oil

Preparation:

Prepare the liver pâté: Wash and finely chop the onion, carrot and celery. Heat the extra virgin olive oil in a pan. Add the chopped vegetables and cook for 3 minutes, stirring occasionally. Add the chicken livers and cook them for 3 minutes over medium heat, stirring often. Add the white wine and cook for another 3 minutes. anchovy, capers, sage, rosemary, salt and pepper to taste. Cook for another 10 minutes over low heat, stirring occasionally.

Remove from the heat and leave to cool. Blend the mixture until you obtain a creamy pâté. Cover with cling film and leave to rest in the refrigerator for at least 15 minutes. Prepare the croutons: Toast the slices of homemade bread in the oven at 180°C for 5-10 minutes, until golden. Brush the toasted bread slices with extra virgin olive oil. Assemble the croutons Spread the liver pâté on the toasted croutons. Serve immediately and enjoy.

Nutritional values (per serving):

Calories: 175 kcal

Fat: 10 g

Carbohydrates: 12 g

Protein: 10 g

Fibres: 1 g

BEEF CARPACCIO

Preparation time: 15 minutes

Cooking time: 0 minutes

Doses: 1 person

Ingredients:

125 g of beef fillet

25 g of wild rocket

25 g of grana padano DOP

Extra virgin olive oil to taste

Lemon juice to taste

Salt and Pepper To Taste

Preparation:

Slice the beef fillet into thin slices (about 2 mm) with a sharp knife. Arrange the slices of meat on a serving plate.

Season with extra virgin olive oil, lemon juice, salt and pepper to taste. Garnish with wild rocket and flaked Grana Padano DOP. Serve immediately and enjoy. For a tastier carpaccio, you can marinate the meat for 15 minutes in an emulsion of extra virgin olive oil, lemon juice, salt, pepper and flavorings to taste.

Nutritional values (per serving):

Calories: 150 kcal

Fat: 7 g

Carbohydrates: 2 g

Protein: 15 g

Fibres: 1 g

SMOKED SALMON CANAPÉS

Preparation time: 10 minutes

Cooking time: 0 minutes

Doses: 1 person

Ingredients:

2 slices of bread for sandwiches

50 g of smoked salmon

25 g of spreadable cheese

(like Philadelphia)

Butter to taste

Pink pepper to taste

Chives to taste

Preparation:

Toast the slices of sandwich bread in the oven at 180°C for 5 minutes, until golden brown. Spread a thin layer of butter on each slice of bread. Spread the spreadable cheese over the bread slices. Add the smoked salmon slices or pieces. Decorate with pink pepper and chopped chives. Serve immediately and enjoy.

Nutritional values (per serving):

Calories: 300 kcal

Fat: 15 g

Carbohydrates: 30 g

Protein: 15 g

Fibers: 2 g

SEAFOOD SALAD

Preparation time: 20 minutes

Cooking time: 10 minutes

(if you use fresh prawns)

Doses: 1 person

Ingredients:

100 g of prawns (fresh or frozen)

50 g of octopus

50 g of calamari

50 g of mussels

50 g of clams

50 g of cherry tomatoes

1/2 red onion

1 cucumber

1/4 of lettuce

Extra virgin olive oil to taste

Lemon juice to taste

Salt and Pepper To Taste

Fresh parsley to taste (optional)

Preparation:

If you use fresh prawns, clean and peel them. Cook the prawns, octopus and squid in boiling salted water for 10 minutes. Open the mussels and clams in a pan with a drizzle of oil and a pinch of white wine. Cut the cherry tomatoes, onion and cucumber into small pieces. Wash the lettuce and cut it into strips. In a large bowl, mix the shrimp, octopus, calamari, mussels, clams, cherry tomatoes, onion, cucumber and lettuce. Season with extra virgin olive oil, lemon juice, salt and pepper to taste.

Decorate with chopped fresh parsley (optional). Serve immediately and enjoy.For a more intense flavour, you can marinate the fish in an emulsion of extra virgin olive oil, lemon juice, aromatic herbs and spices for 30 minutes before cooking it

Nutritional values (per serving):

Calories: 450 kcal

Fat: 20 g

Carbohydrates: 30 g

Protein: 40 g

Fibres: 5 g

HAM AND MELON

Preparation time: 5 minutes

Cooking time: 0 minutes

Doses: 1 person

Ingredients:

150 g of cantaloupe melon

75 g of raw ham

(from Parma or San Daniele)

Fresh mint to taste

Preparation:

Cut the melon into slices about 2 cm thick. Remove the peel and seeds. Cut the raw ham into thin slices.

Arrange the melon slices on a serving plate.
Place the slices of raw ham on the melon.
Garnish with fresh mint leaves. Serve
immediately and enjoy.

Nutritional values (per serving):

Calories: 250 kcal

Fat: 12 g

Carbohydrates: 30 g

Protein: 8 g

Fibers: 2 g

AUBERGINES MEATBALLS

Preparation time: 30 minutes

Cooking time: 20 minutes

Servings: 4 meatballs

Ingredients:

1 medium aubergine

50 g of stale bread

50 g of ricotta

1 egg

2 tablespoons grated parmesan

1 clove of garlic

Fresh basil to taste

Extra virgin olive oil to taste

Salt and Pepper To Taste

Breadcrumbs to taste

Preparation:

Wash the aubergine and cut it into cubes. Fry the aubergine cubes in extra virgin olive oil until golden. Drain them on absorbent paper and let them cool. In a bowl, crumble the stale bread and moisten it with a little milk. Add the ricotta, egg, grated parmesan, chopped garlic, chopped basil, salt and pepper to taste. Mix the mixture well until you obtain a homogeneous mixture. Add the fried aubergines and mix gently. Form meatballs with the mixture obtained and coat them in breadcrumbs. Arrange the meatballs on a baking tray covered with baking paper. Bake in a preheated oven at 180°C for 20 minutes. Serve the aubergine meatballs hot and enjoy. Nutritional values (per serving): Calories: 300 kcal, Fat: 15 g, Carbohydrates: 30 g Protein: 15 g, Fibre: 5 g

ZUCCHINI OMELETTE

Preparation time: 15 minutes

Cooking time: 10 minutes

Doses: 1 person

Ingredients:

2 eggs

1 medium courgette

1 tablespoon of oil

extra virgin olive oil

1 clove of garlic

Salt and Pepper To Taste

Fresh basil to taste (optional)

Preparation:

Wash the courgette and cut it into thin slices. Heat the extra virgin olive oil in a non-stick pan.

Sauté the minced garlic for a minute. Add the courgette slices and cook for 5-7 minutes, stirring occasionally, until softened. In a bowl, beat the eggs with a pinch of salt and pepper. Pour the egg mixture into the pan with the courgettes. Cook the omelette over low heat for 5-7 minutes, until the edges are firm. Fold the omelette in half and cook for another 2 minutes. Serve the courgette omelette hot, garnished with chopped fresh basil (optional).

Nutritional values (per serving):

Calories: 250 kcal

Fat: 15 g

Carbohydrates: 10 g

Protein: 15 g

Fibers: 2 g

RICE ORANGES

Preparation time: 45 minutes

Cooking time: 40 minutes

Doses: 2-3 arancini

Ingredients:

For the rice:

100 g of arborio rice

1/2 onion

1/2 carrot

1/2 stalk of celery

400 ml of vegetable broth

2 tablespoons extra virgin olive oil

1/2 glass of dry white wine

40 g of grated parmesan

Salt and Pepper To Taste

For the stuffing:

50 g of meat sauce

(or other filling to taste)

1 egg Breadcrumbs to taste

Frying oil to taste

Preparation:

Prepare the rice: Finely chop the onion, carrot and celery. Heat the extra virgin olive oil in a saucepan. Fry the chopped vegetables for 5 minutes. Add the rice and toast it for 2 minutes. Add the white wine and cook for 1 minute. Add the vegetable broth one ladle at a time, stirring often, and cook for 15-20 minutes, until the rice is cooked and creamy. Remove from the heat and stir in the grated parmesan, salt and pepper to taste. Allow the rice to cool completely.

Prepare the filling: Mix the meat sauce (or other filling to taste) with the egg. Assemble the arancini: Take a portion of cold rice and shape it into a ball. Make a hole in the center of the rice ball and insert a teaspoon of filling. Close the hole well and give the arancini a round shape. Coat the arancini in breadcrumbs. Fry the arancini: Heat the frying oil in a deep pan. Fry the arancini a few at a time for 4-5 minutes, until they are golden on all sides. Drain them on absorbent paper and serve them hot.

Nutritional values (per serving):

Calories: 500 kcal

Fat: 25 g

Carbohydrates: 10 g

Protein: 15 g

Fibers: 2 g

PRAWNS IN PINK SAUCE

Preparation time: 20 minutes

Cooking time: 10 minutes

Doses: 1 person

Ingredients:

For the pink sauce:

50 g of mayonnaise

1 tablespoon ketchup

1 teaspoon sweet mustard

1 teaspoon Worcestershire sauce

50 ml of fresh cream

Salt and Pepper To Taste

For the shrimp:

200 g of fresh prawns

1 lemon, Water to taste

Salt to taste Pepper to taste

Preparation:

For the pink sauce: In a bowl, mix the mayonnaise, ketchup, sweet mustard, brandy (if using), Worcestershire sauce and fresh cream. Season with salt and pepper to taste. Cover the bowl with cling film and leave to rest in the refrigerator for at least 30 minutes. For the prawns: Wash the prawns and shell them, removing the carapace and the intestinal thread. In a saucepan, bring water to the boil with a pinch of salt. Add the prawns and cook for 3-4 minutes, until pink.

Drain the prawns and let them cool. Drizzle the shrimp with a drizzle of lemon juice. Assemble the dish: Arrange the prawns on a serving plate. Serve the pink sauce separately or pour it over the prawns.

Nutritional values (per serving):

Calories: 350 kcal

Fat: 20 g

Carbohydrates: 5 g

Protein: 30 g

Fibres: 1 g

OLIVE FOCACCIA

Preparation time: 1 hour and 30 minutes

Cooking time: 20 minutes

Doses: 1 small tray

(approximately 20cm in diameter)

Ingredients:

200 g of 00 flour

100 ml of warm water

3 g of fresh brewer's yeast

1 tablespoon extra virgin olive oil

5 g of salt

10 pitted black olives

Rosemary to taste

Preparation:

In a large bowl, dissolve the brewer's yeast in the warm water. Add the flour, extra virgin olive oil and salt. Knead for about 10 minutes, until you obtain a smooth and elastic dough. Cover the bowl with a damp cloth and leave to rise in a warm place for 1 hour. Take the dough and roll it out on an oiled baking tray, forming a disc of about 20 cm in diameter. Poke holes in the surface of the dough with your fingers. Spread the black olives on the focaccia and press them lightly into the dough. Sprinkle the focaccia with a pinch of rosemary.

Cover the pan again with the cloth and leave to rise for another 30 minutes. Cook the focaccia in a preheated oven at 200°C for approximately 20 minutes, until golden. Remove the focaccia from the oven and let it cool slightly before serving.

Nutritional values (per serving):

Calories: 300 kcal

Fat: 15 g

Carbohydrates: 35 g

Protein: 10 g

Fibers: 3 g

MUSHROOMS PIE

Preparation time: 30 minutes

Cooking time: 40 minutes

Doses: 1 small savory pie

(approximately 20cm in diameter)

Ingredients:

For the shortcrust pastry:

150 g of 00 flour

75 g cold butter diced

50 g of grated parmesan

1 egg

A pinch of salt

For the stuffing:

200 g of mixed mushrooms

(champignons, porcini mushrooms, nails)

1 small onion 1 clove of garlic

2 tablespoons extra virgin olive oil

50 ml of fresh cream

2 tablespoons chopped parsley

Salt and Pepper To Taste

Preparation:

For the shortcrust pastry: In a large bowl, mix the flour, grated parmesan and salt. Add the cold diced butter and work the mixture with your fingers until you obtain a sandy dough. Add the egg and mix everything until you obtain a homogeneous mixture. Form the dough into a ball, wrap it in cling film and let it rest in the fridge for 30 minutes. For the filling: Clean the mushrooms and cut them into slices. Finely chop the onion and garlic. Heat the extra virgin olive oil in a pan and fry the onion and garlic for 2-3 minutes. Add the mushrooms and cook them for 10-15 minutes, stirring occasionally, until they are well wilted. Salt and pepper to taste.

Add the fresh cream and chopped parsley and cook for another 2-3 minutes. Remove from the heat and leave to cool. Assemble the savory cake: Preheat the oven to 180°C. Roll out the shortcrust pastry on a sheet of baking paper, forming a disc of about 25 cm in diameter. Transfer the shortcrust pastry disc with the baking paper to a baking tray. Spread the mushroom filling over the shortcrust pastry, leveling it well. Fold the edges of the pastry inwards, creating a decorative edge. Bake in preheated oven for 40 minutes, until golden brown. Remove the savory pie from the oven and let it cool slightly before serving. Nutritional values (per serving):

Calories: 450 kcal

Fat: 25 g

Carbohydrates: 35 g

Protein: 20 g

Fibres: 5 g

HAM AND ASPARAGUS ROLLS

Preparation time: 15 minutes

Cooking time: 10 minutes

Doses: 4 rolls

Ingredients:

4 slices of raw ham

8 asparagus

1 tablespoon extra virgin olive oil

Salt and Pepper To Taste

Preparation:

Wash the asparagus and cut the hard end part. Steam the asparagus for 5-10 minutes, until tender. Arrange a slice of raw ham on a work surface.

Place 2 asparagus on the raw ham. Roll the raw ham on the asparagus, forming a roll. Secure the roll with a toothpick. Repeat the operation for the other 3 rolls. Heat the extra virgin olive oil in a non-stick pan. Cook the ham and asparagus rolls for 2-3 minutes per side, until the ham is golden. Salt and pepper to taste.

Nutritional values (per serving):

Calories: 350 kcal

Fat: 20 g

Carbohydrates: 30 g

Protein: 10 g

Fibres: 5 g

POTATO AND CHEESE PIE

Preparation time: 30 minutes

Cooking time: 40 minutes

Servings: 1 cake

Ingredients:

500 g of potatoes

100 g of grated cheese

(like fontina or provola)

2 eggs

50 ml of milk

2 tablespoons butter

Salt and Pepper To Taste

Breadcrumbs to taste

Preparation:

Peel the potatoes and cut them into thin slices. In a bowl, beat the eggs with the milk, salt and pepper. Add the grated cheese and mix well. Butter a baking tray. Arrange the potato slices in layers in the pan, sprinkling them with the egg and cheese mixture. Sprinkle each layer of potatoes with a little breadcrumbs. Finish with a layer of potatoes and breadcrumbs. Bake in a preheated oven at 180°C for 40 minutes, until golden. Remove the potato and cheese pie from the oven and let it cool slightly before serving. Nutritional values (per serving):

Calories: 550 kcal Fat: 35 g

Carbohydrates: 45 g Proteins: 20 g

Fibres: 5 g

CROSTINI WITH CAPONATA

Preparation time: 20 minutes

Cooking time: 40 minutes

Servings: 4 croutons

Ingredients:

For the caponata:

200 g of aubergines

100 g of peppers (yellow and red)

50 g of celery

50 g of black olives

2 tablespoons of capers

1 small onion

2 cloves of garlic

2 tablespoons extra virgin olive oil

1 tablespoon white wine vinegar

Salt and Pepper To Taste

For the croutons:

4 slices of homemade bread

1 tablespoon extra virgin olive oil

Preparation:

For the caponata: Cut the aubergines into cubes and place them in salted water for 30 minutes. Cut the peppers into strips, the celery into pieces and the olives into slices. Finely chop the onion and garlic cloves. Heat the extra virgin olive oil in a large pan. Saute the onion and garlic for 2-3 minutes. Add the peppers and cook for 10 minutes. Add the drained aubergines and capers and cook for another 10 minutes. Add the black olives and celery and cook for another 5 minutes. Add the white wine vinegar and cook for another 2 minutes. Salt and pepper to taste. Leave the caponata to cool.

For the croutons: Toast the slices of homemade bread in a preheated oven at 180°C for 5 minutes. Brush the toasted bread slices with extra virgin olive oil. Distribute the caponata on the croutons. Serve the crostini with caponata hot or at room temperature.

Nutritional values (per serving):

Calories: 300 kcal

Fat: 20 g

Carbohydrates: 30 g

Protein: 10 g

Fibres: 5 g

MOZZARELLA AND TOMATO SKEWERS

Preparation time: 10 minutes

Cooking time: 0 minutes

Doses: 1 person

Ingredients:

12 cherry tomatoes

8 cherry mozzarella sticks

10 fresh basil leaves

Extra virgin olive oil to taste

Salt to taste

Preparation:

Wash the cherry tomatoes and cut them in half. Drain the mozzarella. Thread a basil leaf, a cherry tomato and a mozzarella on a skewer alternately. Continue skewering the ingredients until the skewer is complete. Season with a drizzle of extra virgin olive oil and a pinch of salt. Serve the mozzarella and cherry tomato skewers immediately.

Nutritional values (per serving):

Calories: 200 kcal

Fat: 12 g

Carbohydrates: 10 g

Protein: 10 g

Fibers: 2 g

SALTY MUFFINS WITH SPINACH AND FETA

Preparation time: 20 minutes

Cooking time: 20 minutes

Servings: 6 muffins

Ingredients:

200 g of 00 flour

50 g of grated parmesan

1 teaspoon baking powder

Salt and Pepper To Taste

2 eggs

150 ml of milk

50 g of melted butter

200 g of fresh spinach

150 g of crumbled feta

Preparation:

Preheat the oven to 180°C. In a large bowl, mix the flour, grated Parmesan, baking powder, salt and pepper. In another bowl, beat the eggs with the milk and melted butter. Add the liquids to the solids and mix until smooth. Add the washed and squeezed spinach and the crumbled feta. Pour the mixture into 6 buttered and floured muffin molds. Bake in preheated oven for 20 minutes, until golden brown. Remove the savory muffins with spinach and feta from the oven and let them cool slightly before serving.

Nutritional values (per serving - 1 muffin):

Calories: 300 kcal

Fat: 15 g

Carbohydrates: 30 g

Protein: 15 g

Fibres: 5 g

STUFFED COURGETTES

Preparation time: 20 minutes

Cooking time: 40 minutes

Doses: 1 person

Ingredients:

2 medium courgettes

100 g minced meat (beef or veal)

50 g of breadcrumbs

25 g of grated parmesan

1/2 egg

1/2 small onion

1 clove of garlic

1 tablespoon extra virgin olive oil

25 ml of tomato sauce

Salt and Pepper To Taste

Preparation:

Wash the courgettes and cut them in half lengthwise, obtaining 2 boats. Empty the courgette boats with a spoon, removing the pulp and creating a hollow. Finely chop the onion and garlic clove. Heat the extra virgin olive oil in a pan and fry the onion and garlic for 2-3 minutes. Add the minced meat and cook for 5 minutes, crumbling with a wooden spoon. Salt and pepper to taste. Add the chopped courgette pulp, breadcrumbs, grated parmesan and half an egg. Mix the mixture well until you obtain a homogeneous mixture. Fill the courgette boats with the meat mixture. Arrange the stuffed courgettes on a baking tray. Pour the tomato sauce onto the bottom of the pan.

Bake in a preheated oven at 180°C for 40 minutes, covering the pan with foil for the first 20 minutes. Uncover the stuffed courgettes during the last 20 minutes of cooking. Remove the stuffed courgettes from the oven and let them cool before serving. Garnish with fresh basil leaves (optional).

Nutritional values (per serving):

Calories: 225 kcal

Fat: 12.5 g

Carbohydrates: 17.5 g

Protein: 12.5 g

Fibers: 2.5 g

Note:

TUNA TARTARE

Preparation time: 10 minutes

Cooking time: 0 minutes

Doses: 1 person

Ingredients:

100 g of fresh tuna

1/2 lemon

1/2 tablespoon capers

1/4 small shallot

5 pitted black olives

2 tablespoons extra virgin olive oil

Salt and Pepper To Taste

Fresh parsley to taste (optional)

Preparation:

Cut the tuna into very small cubes. Finely chop the shallot and capers. Chop the black olives. In a bowl, mix the tuna, shallot, capers, black olives, extra virgin olive oil, juice of half a lemon, salt and pepper to taste. Cover the bowl with cling film and leave to rest in the refrigerator for at least 30 minutes. Serve the tuna tartare with croutons, crackers or green salad. Garnish with chopped fresh parsley (optional).

Nutritional values (per serving):

Calories: 200 kcal

Fat: 10.5 g

Carbohydrates: 15.5 g

Protein: 10.5 g

Fibers: 2.5 g

MEDITERRANEAN CHICKEN SALAD

Preparation time: 20 minutes

Cooking time: 20 minutes

Doses: 1 person

Ingredients:

150 g of chicken breast

100 g of cherry tomatoes

75 g sweet corn

50 g of black olives

75 g of Emmental cheese

Extra virgin olive oil to taste

1-2 fresh basil leaves

Oregano to taste

Salt and Pepper To Taste

Preparation:

Cook the chicken breast: cut the chicken breast into slices about 1 cm thick. Heat a drizzle of extra virgin olive oil in a non-stick pan and cook the chicken slices for 3-4 minutes per side, over medium-high heat, until golden brown. Salt and pepper to taste. Once cooked, cut the chicken into cubes. Prepare the other ingredients: wash the cherry tomatoes and cut them in half. Dissolve the corn from its preserving liquid. Cut the Emmental cheese into cubes. Rinse the black olives, if necessary. Assemble the salad: in a large bowl, combine the diced chicken, cherry tomatoes, corn, black olives and Emmental cheese.

Season the salad: drizzle the salad with a drizzle of extra virgin olive oil, add a chopped fresh basil leaf and a pinch of oregano. Salt and pepper to taste. Gently stir the salad to combine all the ingredients. Serve the Mediterranean chicken salad immediately, at room temperature.

Nutritional values (per serving):

Calories: 400 kcal

Fat: 25 g

Carbohydrates: 25 g

Protein: 25 g

Fibres: 5 g

SALMON WITH ROAST VEGETABLES

Preparation time: 15 minutes

Cooking time: 25 minutes

Doses: 1 person

Ingredients:

1 slice of fresh salmon (about 150 g)

150 g of mixed vegetables (of your choice, e.g example potatoes, carrots, onions, peppers)

Extra virgin olive oil to taste

Salt and Pepper To Taste

Fresh aromatic herbs to taste

(e.g. rosemary, thyme, basil)

Preparation:

Preheat the oven to 200°C. Wash and cut the vegetables into similar sized pieces.

In a large bowl, mix the vegetables with a drizzle of extra virgin olive oil, salt and pepper to taste. Spread the vegetables on a baking tray lined with baking paper. Place the salmon steak on the vegetables. Season the salmon with a drizzle of extra virgin olive oil, salt, pepper and the chosen fresh aromatic herbs. Bake in the preheated oven for 20-25 minutes, or until the salmon is cooked through and the vegetables are golden brown. Serve the salmon with roasted vegetables hot, accompanied by a side of rice or quinoa if desired.

Nutritional values (per serving):

Calories: 450 kcal

Fat: 20 g

Carbohydrates: 35 g

Protein: 30 g

Fibres: 10 g

ZUCCHINI FRITTERS

Preparation time: 15 minutes

Cooking time: 5 minutes

Doses: 1 person

Ingredients:

1 medium courgette

1 egg

25 g of grated cheese

25 g of 00 flour

25 ml of milk

Salt and Pepper To Taste

Seed oil for frying to taste

Fresh basil to taste (optional)

Preparation:

Wash the courgette and grate it coarsely. In a large bowl,

beat the egg with a pinch of salt and pepper. Add the grated cheese, flour and milk, mixing until you obtain a smooth mixture. Add the grated courgette and mix well. Heat the vegetable oil in a non-stick pan over medium heat. Pour a spoonful of mixture into the pan, forming a pancake of about 5 cm in diameter. Cook the pancake for 2-3 minutes per side, or until golden brown. Drain the pancake on absorbent kitchen paper. Serve the courgette pancake hot, accompanied by tomato sauce or Greek yogurt. Garnish with a fresh basil leaf (optional). Nutritional values (per serving): Calories: 100 kcal

Fat: 5 g

Carbohydrates: 10 g

Protein: 5 g

Fibres: 1 g

RAW HAM WITH
FRESH FIGS

Preparation time: 5 minutes

Cooking time: 0 minutes

Doses: 1 person

Ingredients:

50 g of raw ham

2 fresh figs

2 walnuts

Honey to taste

Preparation:

Wash the figs and cut them in half. Shell the walnuts. Arrange the slices of raw ham on a serving plate. Distribute the figs and walnuts between the ham slices. Drizzle with a drizzle of honey. Serve the raw ham appetizer with fresh figs and walnuts. You can also use other types of fresh fruit, such as melon or grapes. If you prefer, you can replace the walnuts with almonds or pistachios. The raw ham appetizer with fresh figs is a simple and refined dish, perfect for a special occasion.

Nutritional values (per serving):

Calories: 150 kcal

Fat: 7.5 g

Carbohydrates: 10 g

Protein: 7.5 g

Fibres: 1 g

CHICKEN AND VEGETABLE SOUP

Preparation time: 15 minutes

Cooking time: 20 minutes

Doses: 1 person

Ingredients:

350 g of chicken pieces

1/2 carrot

1/2 stick of celery 1/4 of onion

1/4 of a sprig of laurel

1/2 sage leaf

Salt and Pepper To Taste

500 ml of water

25 g of short pasta

Preparation:

Wash the chicken and cut it into pieces. Peel the carrot and cut it into slices. Wash the celery

and cut it into pieces. Peel the onion and cut it into slices. In a large pot, place the chicken, carrot, celery, onion, bay leaf, sage, salt and pepper to taste. Cover with water and bring to a boil. Reduce the heat, cover the pot and cook for about 15 minutes, or until the chicken is cooked. Remove the chicken from the pan and let it cool slightly. Strain the broth and return it to the pot. Add the pasta and cook it according to the cooking time indicated on the package. Shred the chicken and add it to the soup. Mix well and serve the chicken and vegetable soup piping hot. Nutritional values (per serving):

Calories: 200 kcal

Fat: 7.5 g

Carbohydrates: 17.5 g

Protein: 15 g

Fibers: 2.5 g

STEAK WITH SWEET POTATOES

Preparation time: 10 minutes

Cooking time: 25 minutes

Doses: 1 person

Ingredients:

1 beef steak (about 200 g)

1 sweet potato

Extra virgin olive oil to taste

Salt and Pepper To Taste

Fresh rosemary to taste (optional)

Preparation:

Preheat the oven to 200°C. Wash the sweet potato and prick it with a fork. Wrap the sweet potato in foil and bake in the oven for about 25 minutes, or until tender.

In the meantime, heat a drizzle of extra virgin olive oil in a non-stick pan over a high heat. Salt and pepper the steak to taste. Cook steak for 2-3 minutes per side, or until desired doneness. Add fresh rosemary to the pan in the last 30 seconds of cooking (optional). Serve the steak with the baked sweet potato.

Nutritional values (per serving):

Calories: 250 kcal

Fat: 12.5 g

Carbohydrates: 25 g

Protein: 15 g

Fibers: 2.5 g

AVOCADO TOAST

Preparation time: 5 minutes

Cooking time: 0 minutes

Doses: 1 person

Ingredients:

1 slice of wholemeal bread

1/2 ripe avocado

Lemon juice to taste

Salt and Pepper To Taste

Optional:

Poached egg

Chia seeds

Chilli flakes

Sriracha sauce

Preparation:

Toast wholemeal bread. Mash the ripe avocado in a bowl with a fork. Add a drizzle of lemon juice, salt and pepper to taste. Spread the avocado cream on the toast. Garnish with optional ingredients of your choice (poached egg, chia seeds, chili flakes, sriracha sauce). You can also use different types of bread, such as white bread or multigrain bread. If the avocado is not ripe enough, you can make it creamier by adding a spoonful of Greek yogurt or ricotta.

Nutritional values (per serving):

Calories: 250 kcal

Fat: 15 g

Carbohydrates: 20 g

Protein: 10 g

Fibres: 5 g

TUNA SALAD

Preparation time: 10 minutes

Cooking time: 0 minutes

Doses: 1 person

Ingredients:

80 g of tuna in oil

1 tomato

1/2 cucumber

1/4 red onion

1/4 of a ripe avocado

10 black olives

Green salad to taste

Extra virgin olive oil to taste

Balsamic vinegar to taste

Salt and Pepper To Taste

Preparation:

Drain the tuna in oil and crumble it into a bowl. Cut the tomato, cucumber, red onion and avocado into small pieces. Add the black olives and the hand-chopped green salad. Season with extra virgin olive oil, balsamic vinegar, salt and pepper to taste. Mix well and serve the tuna salad. You can vary the ingredients of the tuna salad to your taste, for example adding boiled potatoes, hard-boiled eggs or beans. If you prefer a tastier taste, you can use natural tuna and add a pinch of capers.

Nutritional values (per serving):

Calories: 400 kcal

Fat: 25 g

Carbohydrates: 20 g

Protein: 30 g

Fibres: 5 g

CHICKEN BURGER

Preparation time: 15 minutes

Cooking time: 10 minutes

Doses: 1 person

Ingredients:

125 g of minced chicken

1/2 white onion, chopped

1/4 cup breadcrumbs

1 tablespoon chopped fresh parsley

1 egg

Salt and Pepper To Taste

1 tablespoon extra virgin olive oil

Hamburger bun

For garnish (optional):

Tomato, Lettuce, Onion

Preparation:

In a large bowl, mix the minced chicken, chopped onion, breadcrumbs, parsley, egg, salt and pepper to taste. Form the chicken mixture into a compact burger. Heat the extra virgin olive oil in a non-stick pan over medium heat. Cook the chicken burger for 4-5 minutes per side, or until browned and cooked through. Heat the hamburger bun. Fill the sandwich with the chicken burger, vegetables and sauces of your choice. Serve the chicken burger hot.

Nutritional values (per serving):

Calories: 350 kcal

Fat: 15 g

Carbohydrates: 25 g

Protein: 30 g

Fibers: 2 g

VEGETABLE OMELETTE

Preparation time: 5 minutes

Cooking time: 5 minutes

Doses: 1 person

Ingredients:

2 eggs

1 tablespoon of milk

Salt and Pepper To Taste

1 tablespoon extra virgin olive oil

Vegetables of your choice (e.g. tomatoes, spinach, mushrooms, peppers)

Grated cheese to taste (optional)

Preparation:

In a bowl, beat the eggs with the milk, salt and pepper to taste. Heat the extra virgin olive oil in a non-stick pan over medium heat. Pour the egg mixture into the pan and spread evenly. Add the vegetables of your choice, cut into small pieces. Cook the omelet for 2-3 minutes, or until the edges begin to firm up. Fold the omelet in half or thirds. Cook for an additional minute, if desired. Sprinkle with grated cheese (optional). Serve the vegetable omelette hot. Nutritional values (per serving):

Calories: 250 kcal

Fat: 15 g

Carbohydrates: 5 g

Protein: 20 g

Fibers: 2 g

RECIPES
FIRST DISHES

SPAGHETTI CARBONARA

Preparation time 10 minutes

Cooking time 15 minutes

Dose for 1 Person

Ingredients

100 g of spaghetti

50 g of bacon

1 large egg

20 g of pecorino

grated romano

Salt to taste

Black pepper to taste

Preparation

1. Cook the Pasta: Bring a pan of salted water to the boil and cook the spaghetti until al dente (about 8/10 minutes). 2. Prepare the bacon: Cut the bacon into cubes and brown it in a pan over medium heat until crispy (about 5/7 minutes). There is no need to add oil as the bacon will release its fat. 3. Prepare the Egg Cream: In a bowl, beat the egg with the grated pecorino romano and a pinch of black pepper. Mix well until you obtain a smooth cream. 4. Combine the Ingredients: When the spaghetti is cooked, drain it (reserving a little of the cooking water) and add it to the pan with the bacon. Mix well to blend the flavors. 5. Create the Carbonara: Remove the pan from the heat and add the egg and pecorino cream. Stir quickly to prevent the egg from curdling and becoming an omelette.

If necessary, add a little pasta cooking water to make everything creamier. 6. Serve: Serve the spaghetti carbonara immediately, with a sprinkle of black pepper and, if desired, a little additional grated pecorino.

Nutritional Values (per serving)

Calories: 450 kcal Carbohydrates: 50 g Protein: 20 g Fat: 18 g Saturated fat: 6 g Cholesterol: 220 mg Sodium: 600 mg Fibre: 2 g Sugars: 2 g

This classic recipe is simple but full of flavor, perfect for a quick and delicious meal.

ZUCCHINI SPAGHETTI WITH SPINACH PESTO AND CHICKEN

Preparation time: 20 minutes

Cooking time: 15 minutes

Ingredient:

Serves 4 people

4 courgettes

200g chicken breast, cut into cubes

100 g of fresh spinach

30 g of walnuts, 2 cloves of garlic

50 g grated Parmesan

Juice of 1/2 citron

3 tablespoons olive oil, Salt and pepper to taste.

Preparation:

Using a spiralizer or potato peeler, create zucchini "spaghetti". Set them aside. In a pan, heat a tablespoon of olive oil and cook the chicken cubes until cooked through and golden brown. Set it aside. In a blender or blender, combine spinach, walnuts, garlic, grated Parmesan, lemon juice, salt and pepper. Blend until you obtain a creamy consistency. Gradually add olive oil until desired consistency is achieved. In a pan, heat the courgette "spaghetti" with a spoonful of olive oil until tender. Add the spinach pesto to the pan with the courgette "spaghetti" and mix well to season the spaghetti. Add the cooked chicken to the skillet and stir gently. Serve the zucchini "spaghetti" with spinach and chicken pesto. Nutritional values (per serving):

Calories: 400 kcal, Fat: 20 g

Carbohydrates: 50 g, Protein: 10 g Fibre: 2 g

MUSHROOM RISOTTO

Preparation time: 20 minutes

Cooking time: 25 minutes

Doses: 1 person

Ingredients:

80 g of Carnaroli rice

200 g of fresh mixed mushrooms

(or 10 g of dried mushrooms)

1/2 chopped shallot

1/2 glass of dry white wine

500 ml of vegetable broth

1 knob of butter

20 g of grated parmesan

Salt and Pepper To Taste

Preparation:

If you use dried mushrooms, soak them in warm water for 15 minutes.

Clean the fresh mushrooms and cut them into small pieces. In a saucepan, melt the butter over medium heat. Fry the chopped shallots for 2-3 minutes. Add the mushrooms and cook for 5-10 minutes, until soft. Pour in the white wine and let the alcohol evaporate. Add the Carnaroli rice and mix well to add flavour. Gradually add the hot vegetable broth, one ladle at a time, stirring constantly. Cook the risotto for about 20 minutes, or until the rice is creamy and al dente. Season with salt and pepper. Remove from the heat and stir in the grated parmesan. Serve the mushroom risotto hot, garnished with chopped fresh parsley (optional). Nutritional values (per serving): Calories: 450 kcal

Fat: 18 g Carbohydrates: 60 g

Protein: 15 g Fibre: 5 g

TRUFFLE TAGLIATELLE

Preparation time: 15 minutes

Cooking time: 15 minutes

Doses: 1 person

Ingredients:

100 g of fresh tagliatelle

20 g of fresh truffle

(or 1 teaspoon grated truffle)

30 g of butter

1/2 chopped shallot

1/4 glass of dry white wine

50 ml of fresh cream

Salt and Pepper To Taste

Preparation:

Clean the fresh truffle and cut it into thin slices. In a saucepan, melt the butter over medium heat.

Fry the chopped shallots for 2-3 minutes. Pour in the white wine and let the alcohol evaporate. Add the fresh cream and mix well. Cook the tagliatelle in boiling salted water for the time indicated on the package. Drain the tagliatelle al dente and pour them into the saucepan with the sauce. Add the fresh or grated truffle and mix gently. Season with salt and pepper. Serve the truffle tagliatelle piping hot.

Nutritional values (per serving):

Calories: 500 kcal

Fat: 25 g

Carbohydrates: 60 g

Protein: 15 g

Fibers: 2 g

PENNE ALL'ARRABBIATA

Preparation time: 15 minutes

Cooking time: 10 minutes

Doses: 1 person

Ingredients:

80 g of penne

2 tablespoons extra virgin olive oil

1 clove of garlic

1 fresh red chili pepper (optional)

400 g of peeled tomatoes, Salt and pepper to taste

Chopped fresh parsley to taste

Preparation:

Boil the water for the pasta. In a nonstick pan, heat the extra virgin olive oil over medium heat. Add the peeled and crushed garlic (and the chilli if you like) and fry

for a minute. Add the peeled tomatoes, crushed with your hands, and cook for about 10 minutes, stirring occasionally. Salt and pepper to taste. When the water boils, add salt and cook the penne for the time indicated on the package. Drain the penne al dente and pour them into the pan with the arrabiata sauce. Mix well to combine everything. Sprinkle with chopped fresh parsley and serve the penne all'arrabiata piping hot.

Nutritional values (per serving):

Calories: 350 kcal

Fat: 12 g

Carbohydrates: 55 g

Protein: 10 g

Fibres: 5 g

GNOCCHI WITH PESTO

Preparation time: 20 minutes

Cooking time: 15 minutes

Doses: 1 person

Ingredients:

200 g of potato gnocchi

50 g of Genoese pesto

2 tablespoons extra virgin olive oil

2 tablespoons grated parmesan

1 tablespoon pine nuts

Fresh basil to taste (optional)

Salt and Pepper To Taste

Preparation:

Boil the water for the pasta. In a large bowl, mix the Genoese pesto with 2 tablespoons of extra virgin olive oil, grated parmesan and pine nuts. Salt and pepper to taste. When the water boils, add salt and cook the gnocchi for the time indicated on the package. Drain the gnocchi al dente and pour them into the bowl with the pesto. Mix everything well. Serve the gnocchi with pesto piping hot, decorated with fresh basil leaves (optional).

Nutritional values (per serving):

Calories: 500 kcal

Fat: 25 g

Carbohydrates: 65 g

Protein: 15 g

Fibres: 5 g

LASAGNA WITH ARTICHOKE AND SPINACH

Preparation time: 45 minutes

Cooking time: 40 minutes

Doses for 2 people:

Ingredients:

250 g of lasagne pasta

4 artichokes

300 g of spinach

1 liter of bechamel

100 g of grated parmesan

50 g of butter

1 shallot

1 clove of garlic

Extra virgin olive oil

Salt and Pepper To Taste

Preparation:

Clean the artichokes and cut them into thin slices. Fry the chopped shallot and chopped garlic in a pan with extra virgin olive oil for 2 minutes. Add the artichokes and cook for 10 minutes, adding a little water if necessary. Salt and pepper. Blanch the spinach in boiling salted water for 2 minutes, then squeeze and chop coarsely. In a baking pan, spread a little béchamel on the bottom. Make a layer of lasagna pasta, then a layer of artichokes, a layer of spinach and a little bechamel. Repeat the layers until the ingredients are used up. Finish with a layer of béchamel and grated parmesan. Bake in a preheated oven at 180°C for 40 minutes. Remove from the oven and let rest for 10 minutes before serving. Nutritional values (per serving):

Calories: 500 kcal, Carbohydrates: 60 g

Protein: 20 g, Fat: 25 g

QUINOA SALAD WITH GRILLED VEGETABLES

Preparation time: 20 minutes

Cooking time: 20 minutes

Doses for 2 people:

Ingredients:

100 g of quinoa

1 courgette

1 red pepper

1 aubergine

1 red onion

50 g of feta

10 cherry tomatoes

Extra virgin olive oil

Salt and Pepper To Taste

Balsamic vinegar (optional)

Preparation:

Rinse the quinoa under running water for 2 minutes. Cook the quinoa in boiling salted water for 15 minutes. Drain the quinoa and let it cool. Cut the vegetables into slices. Grill the vegetables on a hot grill or in a pan with a drizzle of extra virgin olive oil. Cut the feta into cubes. In a bowl, mix the quinoa, grilled vegetables, feta, cherry tomatoes, extra virgin olive oil, salt and pepper. Add balsamic vinegar to taste. Tips: You can add other ingredients to your taste, such as black olives, capers or fresh basil. If you prefer, you can cook the quinoa in the oven at 180°C for 20 minutes. You can replace the feta with ricotta salata or mozzarella. Nutritional values (per serving):

Calories: 400 kcal, Carbohydrates: 40 g

Protein: 20 g, Fat: 20 g

WHOLE WHOLE SPAGHETTI WITH TUNA AND OLIVES

Preparation time: 15 minutes

Cooking time: 10 minutes

Doses for 2 people:

Ingredients:

160 g of wholemeal spaghetti

120 g of tuna in oil

50 g of black olives

2 tablespoons extra virgin olive oil

1 clove of garlic

Salt and Pepper To Taste

Preparation:

Cook the wholemeal spaghetti in plenty of salted water. In the meantime, drain the tuna and rinse the olives. In a pan, heat the extra virgin olive oil and fry the chopped garlic for 1 minute. Add the tuna and olives and cook for 2 minutes. Drain the spaghetti and sauté them in the pan with the tuna and olives for 1 minute. Salt and pepper. Tips: You can add other ingredients to your taste, such as capers, cherry tomatoes or fresh chilli pepper. If you prefer, you can use natural tuna. Nutritional values (per serving):

Calories: 450 kcal

Carbohydrates: 50 g

Protein: 30 g

Fat: 20 g

WHOLE WHOLE TAGLIATELLE WITH SMOKED SALMON AND CREAM CHEESE

Preparation time: 15 minutes

Cooking time: 10 minutes

Doses for 2 people:

Ingredients:

160 g of wholemeal tagliatelle

100 g of smoked salmon

100 g of spreadable cheese

50 ml of fresh cream

1 tablespoon extra virgin olive oil

Salt and Pepper To Taste

Preparation:

Cook the wholemeal tagliatelle in plenty of salted water. Meanwhile, in a pan, heat the extra virgin olive oil and cook the smoked salmon for 2 minutes. Add the cream cheese and fresh cream and cook for 5 minutes, stirring constantly. Salt and pepper. Drain the tagliatelle and sauté them in the pan with the smoked salmon and cream cheese for 1 minute. Tips: You can add other ingredients to your taste, such as chives or pink pepper. If you prefer, you can use cream cheese instead of cream cheese. Nutritional values (per serving):

Calories: 500 kcal

Carbohydrates: 50 g

Protein: 30 g

Fat: 30 g

ORECCHIETTE WITH TURNIP GREENS

Preparation time: 20 minutes

Cooking time: 15 minutes

Doses: 1 person

Ingredients:

150 g of orecchiette

200 g of turnip greens

1 clove of garlic

1 anchovy (optional)

2 tablespoons extra virgin olive oil

Fresh chili pepper to taste (optional)

Salt and Pepper To Taste

Preparation:

Clean the turnip tops and cut them into small pieces. Boil the water for the pasta.

In a non-stick pan, heat the extra virgin olive oil over medium heat. Add the peeled and crushed garlic (and the anchovy if you like it) and fry for a minute. Add the turnip tops and cook them for about 5 minutes, or until they are softened. Season with salt and pepper to taste. Serve the orecchiette with turnip greens piping hot, sprinkled with grated pecorino to taste.

Nutritional values (per serving):

Calories: 500 kcal

Fat: 20 g

Carbohydrates: 70 g

Protein: 15 g

Fibres: 5 g

FISH SOUP

Preparation time: 30 minutes

Cooking time: 40 minutes

Doses: 1 person

Ingredients:

200 g of mixed fish (including: cod,

hake, scampi, prawns, etc.)

1/2 white onion

1 clove of garlic

1 carrot

1 stick of celery

1 tomato

1/2 glass of dry white wine

500 ml of vegetable broth

1 slice of stale bread

Extra virgin olive oil to taste

Chopped fresh parsley to taste

Salt and Pepper To Taste

Preparation:

Clean the fish and cut it into small pieces. In a pan, heat a drizzle of extra virgin olive oil and fry the chopped onion, the peeled and crushed garlic, the carrot and the celery cut into pieces for a couple of minutes. Add the peeled and crushed tomato with your hands and cook for another 5 minutes. Pour in the white wine and let the alcohol evaporate. Add the vegetable broth and bring to the boil. Add the fish and cook for about 20 minutes, or until the fish is cooked. Salt and pepper to taste. In the meantime, toast the slice of bread stale and rub it with a clove of garlic. When the fish is cooked, turn off the heat and add the chopped fresh parsley. Serve the fish soup piping hot with the slice of toasted bread.

Nutritional values (per serving):

Calories: 450 kcal

Fat: 15 g

Carbohydrates: 40 g

Protein: 35 g

Fibres: 5 g

SAFFRON RISOTTO

Preparation time: 20 minutes

Cooking time: 25 minutes

Doses: 1 person

Ingredients:

80 g of Carnaroli rice

1/2 white onion

1/2 sachet of saffron

500 ml of vegetable broth

1 knob of butter

20 g of grated parmesan

Salt and Pepper To Taste

Preparation:

In a saucepan, melt the butter over medium heat. Fry the chopped onion for a couple of minutes.

Add the Carnaroli rice and mix well to flavor it. Dissolve the saffron in a ladle of hot broth and add it to the rice. Add the hot broth, one ladle at a time, stirring constantly. Cook the risotto for about 20 minutes, or until the rice is creamy and al dente. Season with salt and pepper. Remove from the heat and stir in the grated parmesan. Serve the saffron risotto piping hot.

Nutritional values (per serving):

Calories: 450 kcal

Fat: 18 g

Carbohydrates: 60 g

Protein: 15 g

Fibres: 5 g

FETTUCCINE ALFREDO

Preparation time: 15 minutes

Cooking time: 15 minutes

Doses: 1 person

Ingredients:

100 g of fettuccine

50 g of butter

50 g of grated parmesan

1/2 clove of garlic

Salt and Pepper To Taste

Fresh parsley

chopped to taste (optional)

Preparation:

Boil the water for the pasta. In a large skillet, melt the butter over medium heat. Add the peeled and crushed garlic and fry for a minute. Add the fettuccine al dente and mix well to mix them with the butter. Add the grated parmesan, salt and pepper to taste. Mix again to melt the cheese and create a cream. Serve the fettuccine Alfredo piping hot, sprinkled with chopped fresh parsley (optional).

Nutritional values (per serving):

Calories: 500 kcal

Fat: 25 g

Carbohydrates: 60 g

Protein: 15 g

Fibers: 2 g

SPAGHETTI WITH MUSSELS

Preparation time: 20 minutes

Cooking time: 20 minutes

Doses: 1 person

Ingredients:

100 g of spaghetti

200 g of mussels

1 clove of garlic

2 tablespoons extra virgin olive oil

1/2 glass of dry white wine

Chopped fresh parsley to taste

Salt and Pepper To Taste

Preparation:

Clean the mussels and rinse them carefully under running water. Discard any with cracked or open shells. Boil the water for the pasta.

In a non-stick pan, heat the extra virgin olive oil olive oil over medium heat. Add the peeled and crushed garlic (and the chilli if you like) and fry for a minute. Add the mussels and deglaze with the white wine. Cover the pan with a lid and cook for about 5 minutes, or until the mussels have opened. Discard any mussels that have not opened. Dissolve a spoonful of the pasta cooking water in the pan with the mussels to create a sauce. Salt and pepper to taste. When the water boils, add salt and cook the spaghetti for the time indicated on the package. Drain the spaghetti al dente and pour them into the pan with the mussels. Mix well to combine everything. Serve the spaghetti with mussels piping hot, sprinkled with fresh chopped parsley. Nutritional values (per serving): Calories: 450 kcal Fat: 18 g

Carbohydrates: 55 g Protein: 25 g Fibre: 3 g

VEGETABLE MINESTRONE

Preparation time: 30 minutes

Cooking time: 1 hour and 30 minutes

Doses: 1 person

Ingredients:

200 g of mixed vegetables (including: carrots, potatoes, courgettes, green beans, tomatoes, etc.)

1/2 white onion, 1 clove of garlic

1 stick of celery

1 tablespoon extra virgin olive oil

1 liter of vegetable broth

50 g of short pasta

Chopped fresh basil to taste

Salt and Pepper To Taste

Preparation:

Wash and clean the vegetables. Cut the carrots, potatoes and courgettes into small pieces, the green beans in half and the tomatoes into cubes. In a large pot, heat the extra virgin olive oil over medium heat. Fry the chopped onion and the peeled and crushed garlic for a couple of minutes. Add the mixed vegetables and mix well to combine them. Pour in the vegetable broth and bring to the boil. Cook for about 1 hour, or until the vegetables are tender. Add the pasta and cook it for the time indicated on the package. Salt and pepper to taste. At the end of cooking, turn off the heat and add the chopped fresh basil. Serve the vegetable minestrone piping hot. Nutritional values (per serving): Calories: 350 kcal Fat: 12 g

Carbohydrates: 45 g Protein: 15 g Fiber: 5 g

FUSILLI WITH CHEES AND PEPPER

Preparation time: 15 minutes

Cooking time: 15 minutes

Doses: 1 person

Ingredients:

100 g of fusilli

50 g of grated pecorino romano

1/2 teaspoon ground black pepper

2 tablespoons extra virgin olive oil

Pasta cooking water to taste

Preparation:

Boil the water for the pasta. In a large bowl, mix the grated pecorino romano and ground black pepper.

When the water boils, add salt and cook the fusilli for the time indicated on the package. Drain the fusilli al dente, keeping a ladle of the cooking water. Pour the fusilli into the bowl with the pecorino and pepper. Add the cooking water little by little, stirring vigorously, until you create a thick, smooth cream. Add the extra virgin olive oil and mix well. Serve the fusilli cacio e pepe piping hot, stirring once more before enjoying them. Nutritional values (per serving):

Calories: 500 kcal

Fat: 28 g

Carbohydrates: 55 g

Protein: 20 g

Fibers: 2 g

CABBAGE PAD THAI

Preparation time: 20 minutes

Cooking time: 15 minutes

Doses for 2 people:

Ingredients:

150 g of kale

150 g of Thai rice

1 tablespoon extra virgin olive oil

1 red onion

1 red pepper

1 fresh chili pepper

2 eggs

2 tablespoons soy sauce

2 tablespoons lime juice

1 tablespoon brown sugar

1 tablespoon chopped peanuts

Salt and Pepper To Taste

Preparation:

Cut the kale into thin strips. Cook the Thai rice in boiling salted water for 10 minutes. In the meantime, heat the extra virgin olive oil in a pan and fry the chopped onion for 2 minutes. Add the pepper cut into strips and the chopped chilli and cook for 5 minutes. Add the eggs and cook them scrambled. Add the Thai rice, kale, soy sauce, lime juice, brown sugar and chopped peanuts. Salt and pepper. Cook for another 5 minutes, stirring constantly. Nutritional values (per serving):

Calories: 400 kcal

Carbohydrates: 50 g

Protein: 20 g

Fat: 20 g

TOMATO AND BASIL SOUP WITH WHOLEMEAL CROUTTONS

Preparation time: 20 minutes

Cooking time: 30 minutes

Doses for 2 people:

Ingredients:

500 g of peeled tomatoes

1 white onion

2 cloves of garlic

50 g of fresh basil

1 tablespoon extra virgin olive oil

Salt and Pepper To Taste

Whole grain bread

Extra virgin olive oil

Preparation:

In a pan, heat the extra virgin olive oil and fry the chopped onion and garlic chopped for 2 minutes. Add the peeled tomatoes and cook for 20 minutes. Blend the soup with a blender. Add chopped fresh basil, salt and pepper. Cook for another 5 minutes. Cut the wholemeal bread into slices and toast it in the oven with a drizzle of extra virgin olive oil. Serve the tomato and basil soup with wholemeal bread croutons. Tips: You can add other ingredients to your taste, such as chopped vegetables, such as carrots or celery. If you prefer, you can use fresh tomatoes instead of peeled tomatoes. Nutritional values (per serving):

Calories: 200 kcal

Carbohydrates: 25 g

Protein: 5 g

Fat: 10 g

ZUCCHINI TAGLIATELLE WITH PRAWNS AND GARLIC

Preparation time: 15 minutes

Cooking time: 10 minutes

Doses for 2 people:

Ingredients:

2 courgettes

200 g of peeled prawns

2 cloves of garlic

1 tablespoon of oil

extra virgin olive oil

Salt and Pepper To Taste

Fresh parsley to taste

Preparation:

Cut the courgettes into julienne strips with a grater or sharp knife. Clean the prawns and shell them. In a pan, heat the extra virgin olive oil and fry the chopped garlic for 1 minute. Add the prawns and cook for 2 minutes. Add the courgettes and cook for 5 minutes. Salt and pepper. Serve the prawn and garlic courgette tagliatelle with chopped fresh parsley. Tips: You can add other ingredients to your taste, such as cherry tomatoes or fresh chilli pepper. If you prefer, you can use frozen shrimp.

Nutritional values (per serving):

Calories: 250 kcal

Carbohydrates: 10 g

Protein: 30 g

Fat: 10 g

BLACK BEAN SOUP WITH AVOCADO

Preparation time: 20 minutes

Cooking time: 20 minutes

Doses for 2 people:

Ingredients:

250g canned black beans

1 white onion

1 carrots

1 stalk of celery

2 cloves of garlic

1 bay leaf

1 sprig of rosemary

1 tablespoon extra virgin olive oil

Salt and pepper to taste, 1 avocado

Lime juice, fresh coriander to taste

Preparation:

Rinse the beans and place them in a pan with cold water. Add the chopped onion, the diced carrots, the diced celery, the chopped garlic, the bay leaf and the rosemary. Bring to the boil, then reduce the heat and cook for 20 minutes. Blend the soup with a blender. Salt and pepper. Cut the avocado in half, remove the stone and peel. Mash the avocado with a fork and add the lime juice. Serve black bean soup with avocado and chopped fresh cilantro. Tips: You can add other ingredients to your taste, such as fresh chili pepper or paprika. Nutritional values (per serving):

Calories: 300 kcal

Carbohydrates: 30 g

Protein: 15 g

Fat: 15 g

WHOLEMEAL TAGLIATELLE WITH AVOCADO SAUCE AND TOMATOES

Preparation time: 15 minutes

Cooking time: 10 minutes

Doses for 2 people:

Ingredients:

160 g of wholemeal tagliatelle

1 avocado

100 g of cherry tomatoes

1/2 red onion

2 tablespoons extra virgin olive oil

1 tablespoon lemon juice

Salt and Pepper To Taste

Preparation:

Cook the wholemeal tagliatelle in boiling salted water for 8 minutes. In the meantime, prepare the sauce: blend the avocado, cherry tomatoes, red onion, extra virgin olive oil, lemon juice, salt and pepper. Drain the tagliatelle and season them with the avocado sauce. Tips: You can add other ingredients to your taste, such as black olives or fresh basil. If you prefer, you can use peeled tomatoes instead of cherry tomatoes. Nutritional values (per serving):

Calories: 400 kcal

Carbohydrates: 50 g

Protein: 15 g

Fat: 20 g

GREEN BEAN SALAD WITH TUNA AND BOILED EGGS

Preparation time: 15 minutes

Cooking time: 10 minutes

Doses for 2 people:

Ingredients:

200 g of green beans

1 can of tuna 100 g.

2 hard boiled eggs

1 red onion

1 tablespoon extra virgin olive oil

1 tablespoon lemon juice

Salt and Pepper To Taste

Preparation:

Cook the green beans in boiling salted water for 5 minutes. Cut the hard-boiled eggs into small pieces. Cut the red onion into thin slices. In a bowl, mix the green beans, tuna, hard-boiled eggs, red onion, extra virgin olive oil, lemon juice, salt and pepper. Tips: You can add other ingredients to your taste, green olives. If you prefer, you can use frozen green beans instead of fresh green beans. Nutritional values (per serving):

Calories: 300 kcal

Carbohydrates: 20 g

Protein: 30 g

Fat: 15 g

RISOTTO WITH CHICORY AND GORGONZOLA

Preparation time: 15 minutes

Cooking time: 20 minutes

Doses: 1 person

Ingredients:

80 g of Carnaroli rice

1 white onion, 100 g of Chicory

50 g of sweet gorgonzola

50 ml of dry white wine

1/2 liter of vegetable broth

20 g of butter, Salt and pepper to taste

Preparation:

Clean and chop the onion. Cut the radicchio into strips. In a large saucepan, melt the butter over medium heat. Add the chopped

onion and fry for a couple of minutes, until tender transparent. Add the radicchio cut into strips and cook for 5 minutes, stirring often. Pour in the white wine and let the alcohol evaporate. Add the Carnaroli rice and mix well to add flavour. Salt and pepper to taste. Pour the vegetable broth one ladle at a time, stirring constantly. Cook the risotto for about 20 minutes, or until the rice is creamy and al dente. Turn off the heat and add the sweet gorgonzola cut into cubes. Mix well until the cheese has melted and created a cream. Serve the radicchio and gorgonzola risotto piping hot. Nutritional values (per serving):

Calories: 550 kcal Fat: 28 g

Carbohydrates: 65 g Proteins: 20 g

Fibres: 5 g

SPAGHETTI WITH GARLIC, OIL AND CHILI PEPPER

Preparation time: 10 minutes

Cooking time: 10 minutes

Doses: 1 person

Ingredients:

100 g of spaghetti

2 cloves of garlic

1 fresh chili pepper (optional)

4 tablespoons of extra virgin olive oil

Salt and Pepper To Taste

Chopped fresh parsley to taste

Preparation:

Boil the water for the pasta. In a large skillet, heat the extra virgin olive oil over medium heat. Fry the peeled and crushed garlic for a minute, until golden.

Add the chopped fresh chilli (if desired) and mix to flavor the oil. Salt and pepper to taste. When the water boils, add salt and cook the spaghetti for the time indicated on the package. Drain the spaghetti al dente and pour them into the pan with the oil, garlic and chilli. Mix well to combine everything. Add the chopped fresh parsley and serve the spaghetti with garlic, oil and chilli hot.

Nutritional values (per serving):

Calories: 462 kcal

Fat: 17.8 g

Carbohydrates: 66.7 g

Protein: 8.7 g

Fibers: 2.2 g

GREEK PASTA SALAD

Preparation time: 20 minutes

Cooking time: 15 minutes

Doses: 1 person

Ingredients:

100 g of pasta (penne, farfalle or fusilli)

1/2 cucumber

1/2 tomato

1/4 red onion

100 g of feta

10 black olives

2 tablespoons extra virgin olive oil

1 tablespoon lemon juice

Dried oregano to taste

Salt and Pepper To Taste

Preparation:

Cook the pasta in plenty of salted water for the time indicated on the package. Drain it al dente and cool it under running water. Cut the cucumber, tomato and red onion into small pieces. Crumble the feta and pit the black olives. In a large bowl, mix the chilled pasta, cucumber, tomato, red onion, feta and black olives. Season with extra virgin olive oil, lemon juice, dried oregano, salt and pepper to taste. Mix well and serve the fresh Greek pasta salad.

Nutritional values (per serving):

Calories: 450 kcal

Fat: 20 g

Carbohydrates: 55 g

Protein: 20 g

Fibres: 5 g

PASTA WITH GENOESE PESTO

Preparation time: 15 minutes

Cooking time: 10 minutes

Doses: 1 person

Ingredients:

100 g of pasta (trofie, Genoese or linguine)

50 g of Genoese pesto

30 g of grated parmesan

2 tablespoons extra virgin olive oil

Fresh basil to decorate (optional)

Salt and Pepper To Taste

Preparation:

Boil the water for the pasta. In a large bowl, mix the Genoese pesto with the grated parmesan and a spoon

of extra virgin olive oil. Salt and pepper to taste. When the water boils, add salt and cook the pasta for the time indicated on the package. Drain the pasta al dente and season it with the prepared pesto, mixing well to combine everything. Add another tablespoon of extra virgin olive oil if necessary. Serve the pasta with pesto piping hot, decorating with fresh basil leaves (optional).

Nutritional values (per serving):

Calories: 500 kcal

Fat: 25 g

Carbohydrates: 65 g

Protein: 15 g

Fibres: 5 g

MUSHROOM RISOTTO

Preparation time: 20 minutes

Cooking time: 25 minutes

Doses: 1 person

Ingredients:

80 g of Carnaroli rice

1/2 white onion

200 g of mixed mushrooms

(porcini mushrooms, mushrooms, tacks)

1/2 glass of dry white wine

500 ml of vegetable broth

1 knob of butter

30 g of grated parmesan

Chopped fresh parsley to taste

Salt and Pepper To Taste

Preparation:

Clean the mushrooms and cut them into small pieces. In a saucepan, heat the butter over medium heat. Fry the chopped onion for a couple of minutes. Add the mushrooms and cook for 5 minutes, stirring often. Pour in the white wine and let the alcohol evaporate. Add the Carnaroli rice and mix well to add flavour. Salt and pepper to taste. Pour the vegetable broth one ladle at a time, stirring constantly. Cook the risotto for about 20 minutes, or until the rice is creamy and al dente. Turn off the heat and add the grated parmesan and chopped fresh parsley. Mix well and serve the mushroom risotto piping hot. Nutritional values (per serving):

Calories: 450 kcal Fat: 18 g

Carbohydrates: 60 g Protein: 15 g Fibre: 5 g

PENNE WITH TOMATO AND BASIL

Preparation time: 20 minutes

Cooking time: 30 minutes

Doses: 1 person

Ingredients:

100 g of penne

400 g of peeled tomatoes

1/2 white onion

1 clove of garlic

2 tablespoons extra virgin olive oil

Chopped fresh basil to taste

Salt and Pepper To Taste

Grated parmesan to taste (optional)

Preparation:

In a large skillet, heat the extra virgin olive oil over medium heat.

Fry the chopped onion and the peeled and crushed garlic for a couple of minutes. Add the peeled tomatoes crushed with your hands and a pinch of salt. Cook the tomato sauce for about 20 minutes, stirring occasionally. Add the chopped fresh basil and mix. Salt and pepper to taste. In the meantime, cook the penne in plenty of salted water for the time indicated on the package. Drain the penne al dente and pour it into the pan with the tomato sauce. Stir gently to combine everything. Serve the penne with tomato and basil piping hot. Nutritional values (per serving):

Calories: 450 kcal Fat: 15 g

Carbohydrates: 65 g Proteins: 15 g

Fibres: 5 g

SPAGHETTI ALLA MATRICIANA

Preparation time: 25 minutes

Cooking time: 20 minutes

Doses: 1 person

Ingredients:

100 g of spaghetti

150 g of pork cheek

1/2 white onion

1 clove of garlic

70 ml of dry white wine

400 g of peeled tomatoes

Grated pecorino romano to taste

Salt and Pepper To Taste

Preparation:

Cut the pork cheek into small pieces. In a large skillet, heat a drizzle of olive oil over medium heat. Fry the onion

chopped and the garlic peeled and crushed for a couple of minutes. Add the bacon and cook until crispy. Pour in the white wine and let the alcohol evaporate. Add the peeled tomatoes crushed with your hands and a pinch of salt. Cook the sauce for about 15 minutes, stirring occasionally. In the meantime, cook the spaghetti in plenty of salted water for the time indicated on the package. Drain the spaghetti al dente and pour them into the pan with the sauce. Mix well to combine everything. Add the grated pecorino romano to taste and mix. Serve the spaghetti matriciana piping hot, with a sprinkling of grated pecorino romano. Nutritional values (per serving): Calories: 650 kcal Fat: 35 g

Carbohydrates: 70 g Protein: 30 g Fibre: 5 g

RECIPES
SECOND DISHES

BAKED SEA BASS

Preparation time: 20 minutes

Cooking time: 20-25 minutes

Doses: 1 person

Ingredients:

1 fresh sea bass, 300 g

Extra virgin olive oil to taste

Lemon to taste

Salt to taste

Tomatoes to taste (optional)

Black olives to taste (optional)

**Fresh aromatic herbs a
pleasure (rosemary, thyme, sage)**

Preparation:

**Clean the sea bass: Gut the sea bass and
scale it. Wash it thoroughly underneath**

running water and dry it with kitchen paper. Season the sea bass: In a bowl, drizzle the sea bass with extra virgin olive oil, salt and freshly ground black pepper. Add the juice of one lemon and fresh herbs to taste. Arrange the sea bass on a baking tray: Place the sea bass on a bed of new potatoes, cherry tomatoes and black olives (optional). Cook in the oven: Bake the sea bass in a preheated oven at 180°C for 20-25 minutes, or until cooking is complete (the fish flesh must be white and compact). Serve: Remove the sea bass from the oven and serve hot with the new potatoes, cherry tomatoes and black olives (if used). Nutritional values (per serving): Calories: 450 kcal Fat: 25 g

Protein: 60 g Carbohydrates: 10 g

Fibers: 2 g

GRILLED SWORDFISH

Preparation time: 15 minutes

Cooking time: 10 minutes

Doses: 1 person

Ingredients:

1 swordfish steak weighing 200-250 g

Extra virgin olive oil to taste

Lemon to taste

Salt to taste

Freshly ground black pepper to taste

Rosemary to taste (optional)

Preparation:

Clean the swordfish: Carefully wash the swordfish steak under running water and dry it with kitchen paper. Season the swordfish:

In a bowl, drizzle the swordfish with extra virgin olive oil, salt and freshly ground black pepper. Add the juice of one lemon and the rosemary (optional). Grill swordfish: Heat a grill over medium-high heat. Lightly grease the grill with extra virgin olive oil. Place the swordfish steak on the grill and cook for 4-5 minutes per side, or until golden and firm. Serve: Remove the grilled swordfish from the oven and serve hot with a side of grilled vegetables or a fresh salad. Nutritional values (per serving):

Calories: 400 kcal

Fat: 20 g

Protein: 50 g

Carbohydrates: 10 g

Fibers: 2 g

POTATO OMELETTE

Preparation time: 15 minutes

Cooking time: 10 minutes

Doses: 1 person

Ingredients:

100 g of potatoes

2 eggs

1/2 white onion (optional)

30 g of grated parmesan

Extra virgin olive oil to taste

Salt to taste

Freshly ground black pepper to taste

Preparation:

Peel the potatoes and cut them into cubes of about 1 cm. In a non-stick pan, heat a drizzle of extra virgin olive oil and fry the finely chopped onion (if used).

Add the diced potatoes and cook for about 10 minutes, stirring occasionally, until they are soft. In a bowl, beat the eggs with the grated parmesan, salt and pepper. Pour the cooked potatoes and chopped parsley (if using) into the egg mixture and mix well. Heat a drizzle of extra virgin olive oil in a non-stick pan with a diameter of approximately 15 cm. Pour the egg and potato mixture into the pan and cook over medium-low heat for about 5 minutes, or until the omelette is well set on the bottom. With the help of a plate, turn the omelette over and cook it for another 2-3 minutes on the other side. Peel the potato omelette and serve it hot.

Nutritional values (per serving):

Calories: 350 kcal Fat: 15 g

Protein: 15 g Carbohydrates: 40 g Fiber: 5 g

BEEF FILLET WITH GREEN PEPPER

Preparation time: 20 minutes

Cooking time: 10 minutes

Doses: 1 person

Ingredients:

200 g of beef fillet

1 tablespoon green peppercorns

1/2 shallot

100 ml of fresh cream

Butter to taste

Extra virgin olive oil to taste

Salt to taste

Freshly ground black pepper to taste

Preparation:

Crush the green peppercorns with a mortar.
Finely chop the shallot.

In a pan, heat a drizzle of oil extra virgin olive oil and brown the beef fillet on all sides to seal it. Add the butter, chopped shallots and crushed green pepper. Cook the beef tenderloin for 5-7 minutes per side, or until desired doneness. Add a ladle of hot water and cook for a couple of minutes. Add the fresh cream, salt and pepper. Cook for another minute, stirring, until you get a creamy sauce. Serve the beef fillet with green pepper piping hot with its sauce. Nutritional values (per serving):

Calories: 450 kcal

Fat: 10 g

Protein: 15 g

Carbohydrates: 30 g

Fibers: 2 g

GRILLED CHICKEN WITH MIXED VEGETABLES

Preparation time: 20 minutes

Cooking time: 20 minutes

Doses for 2 people

Ingredients:

2 chicken breasts

1 courgette

1 red pepper

1 aubergine

1 red onion

2 tablespoons of oil

extra virgin olive oil

Salt and Pepper To Taste

Preparation:

Cut the chicken into slices about 2cm thick. Wash the vegetables and cut them into slices. In a bowl, mix the extra virgin olive oil with salt and pepper. Marinate the chicken and vegetables in the bowl for 15 minutes. Heat a grill over medium-high heat. Cook the chicken and vegetables for about 20 minutes, turning them halfway through cooking. Serve the chicken with the grilled vegetables. Nutritional values (per serving):

Calories: 350

Fat: 15 g

Protein: 40 g

Carbohydrates: 10 g

BAKED SALMON WITH ASPARAGUS

Preparation time: 15 minutes

Cooking time: 20 minutes

Doses for 2 people

Ingredients:

2 salmon fillets

100 g of asparagus

1 tablespoon of oil

extra virgin olive oil

Salt and Pepper To Taste

1 lemon

Preparation:

Preheat the oven to 180°C. Wash the asparagus and cut off the tough end part. Arrange the salmon fillets on a baking tray. Season the salmon with extra virgin olive oil, salt and pepper. Arrange the asparagus around the salmon. Bake in the oven for 20 minutes. Serve the salmon with the asparagus and drizzle with the juice of a lemon.

Nutritional values (per serving):

Calories: 400

Fat: 20 g

Protein: 45 g

Carbohydrates: 5 g

BEEF STEAK WITH
GREEN PEPPER SAUCE

Preparation time: 30 minutes

Cooking time: 20 minutes

Doses for 2 people

Ingredients:

2 beef steaks, 200g each

2 tablespoons pickled green pepper

1/2 glass of fresh cream

1 tablespoon brandy

1 tablespoon butter

Salt and Pepper To Taste

Preparation:

Rinse the beef steaks and dry them with kitchen paper. Crush the green peppercorns with a mortar. In a nonstick skillet, melt the butter over medium-high heat. Cook steaks for 4-5 minutes per side, or until desired doneness. Remove the steaks from the pan and keep warm. In the same pan, add the green pepper and brandy. Cook for 1 minute, stirring with a wooden spoon. Add the fresh cream and cook for a further 5 minutes, or until the sauce has thickened. Salt and pepper to taste. Serve the steaks with the green pepper sauce. Nutritional values (per serving):

Calories: 500

Fat: 30 g

Protein: 40 g

Carbohydrates: 5 g

FISH FILLET WITH

LEMON AND PARSLEY

Preparation time: 15 minutes

Cooking time: 15 minutes

Doses for 2 people

Ingredients:

2 white fish fillets

(cod, trout, sea bream, etc.)

1 lemon

1 tablespoon chopped parsley

1 tablespoon of oil

extra virgin olive oil

Salt and Pepper To Taste

Preparation:

Preheat the oven to 180°C. Wash the lemon and cut it into thin slices. Rinse the fish fillets and dry them with kitchen paper. Arrange the fish fillets on a baking tray. Season the fish with extra virgin olive oil, salt and pepper. Distribute the lemon slices and chopped parsley over the fish fillets. Bake in the oven for 15 minutes. Serve the fish with the lemon and parsley sauce.

Nutritional values (per serving):

Calories: 250

Fat: 10 g

Protein: 35 g

Carbohydrates: 5 g

TURKEY MEATBALLS WITH TOMATO SAUCE

Preparation time: 30 minutes

Cooking time: 30 minutes

Doses for 2 people

Ingredients:

250 g of minced turkey

1 egg

50 g of grated parmesan

50 g of breadcrumbs

1 white onion

1 carrot

1 stalk of celery

200 g of peeled tomatoes

1 tablespoon extra virgin olive oil

Salt and Pepper To Taste

Preparation:

In a large bowl, mix the ground turkey with the egg, grated parmesan, breadcrumbs, salt and pepper. Finely chop the onion, carrot and celery. In a non-stick pan, heat the extra virgin olive oil and fry the chopped vegetables for 5 minutes. Add the peeled tomatoes and cook for 15 minutes, stirring occasionally. Salt and pepper to taste. Form meatballs with the ground turkey mixture. Add the meatballs to the tomato sauce and cook for another 15 minutes. Serve the meatballs with the tomato sauce. Nutritional values (per serving):

Calories: 400

Fat: 20 g

Protein: 30 g

Carbohydrates: 20 g

CHICKEN BREAST STUFFED WITH CHEESE AND SPINACH

Preparation time: 20 minutes

Cooking time: 30 minutes

Doses for 2 people

Ingredients:

2 chicken breasts

100 g of spinach

50 g of ricotta

50 g of grated parmesan

1 white onion

1 clove of garlic

1 tablespoon of oil

extra virgin olive oil

Salt and Pepper To Taste

Preparation:

Open the chicken breasts like a book and beat them with a meat mallet. In a non-stick pan, heat the extra virgin olive oil and fry the chopped onion and chopped garlic for 5 minutes. Add the spinach and cook for 5 minutes, stirring occasionally. Salt and pepper to taste. In a bowl, mix the ricotta, grated parmesan and sautéed spinach. Stuff the chicken breasts with the ricotta and spinach mixture. Close the chicken breasts with toothpicks. Arrange the stuffed chicken breasts on a baking tray. Bake in a preheated oven at 180°C for 30 minutes. Serve the stuffed chicken breasts hot. Nutritional values (per serving):

Calories: 450, Fat: 25 g

Protein: 40 g

Carbohydrates: 10 g

GRILLED SWORDFISH

Preparation time: 15 minutes

Cooking time: 10 minutes

Doses: 1 person

Ingredients:

200-250 g of swordfish steak

Extra virgin olive oil to taste

Lemon to taste

Salt to taste

Freshly ground black pepper to taste

Rosemary to taste (optional)

Preparation:

Clean the swordfish: Carefully wash the swordfish steak under running water and dry it with kitchen paper. Season the swordfish: In a bowl, drizzle the swordfish with extra virgin olive oil, salt and

freshly ground black pepper. Add the juice of one lemon and the rosemary (optional). Grill swordfish: Heat a grill over medium-high heat. Lightly grease the grill with extra virgin olive oil. Place the swordfish steak on the grill and cook for 4-5 minutes per side, or until golden and firm. Serve: Remove the grilled swordfish from the oven and serve hot with a side of grilled vegetables or a fresh salad. If you like, you can squeeze a little lemon juice on the swordfish before serving. Nutritional values (per serving):

Calories: 350 kcal

Fat: 20 g

Protein: 50 g

Carbohydrates: 5 g

Fibres: 1 g

ESCALLOPPINE WITH LEMON

Preparation time: 20 minutes

Cooking time: 10 minutes

Doses: 1 person

Ingredients:

200 g of veal slices

(thinly cut and beaten)

1 lemon

Flour to taste

Butter to taste

Salt to taste

Freshly ground black pepper to taste

Preparation:

Flour the veal slices: Place the flour on a flat plate and carefully flour the veal slices on both sides, eliminating any excess.

Flour. Melt the butter: In a large skillet, heat the butter over medium-high heat. If you prefer a lighter flavour, you can use a drizzle of extra virgin olive oil instead of butter. Cook the scallops: Place the floured veal slices in the pan with the melted butter and cook them for about 2-3 minutes on each side, or until golden brown. Add the lemon: Squeeze the juice of a lemon onto the scallops and cook for another minute, stirring gently to mix the juice with the butter. Salt and pepper: Add salt and freshly ground black pepper to taste. Serve: Plate the scallops with lemon and garnish with chopped fresh parsley (optional). Serve hot with a side of baked potatoes or grilled vegetables. Nutritional values (per serving): Calories: 350 kcal Fat: 25 g Protein: 30 g Carbohydrates: 5 g Fibre: 1 g

VENETIAN STYLE LIVER

Preparation time: 20 minutes

Cooking time: 20 minutes

Doses: 1 person

Ingredients:

300 g of calf liver

(cut into thin slices)

2 medium white onions

1 tablespoon extra virgin olive oil

1 knob of butter

2 tablespoons white wine vinegar

1 tablespoon chopped parsley

Salt to taste

Freshly ground black pepper to taste

Flour to taste (optional)

Preparation:

Clean the liver: Wash the calf liver carefully under running water and dry it with kitchen paper. Remove any films or ribs. If necessary, cut the liver into thin slices about 1 cm thick. Flour the liver (optional): If you want a crispier breading, lightly flour the liver slices on both sides. Sauté the onions: In a large skillet, heat the extra virgin olive oil over medium heat. Finely slice the onions and add them to the pan. Fry the onions for about 15 minutes, stirring occasionally, until they are well wilted and golden. Add the liver: Add the floured liver slices (if using flour) to the fried onions. Salt and pepper to taste. Deglaze with vinegar: Deglaze the liver with white wine vinegar, stirring gently to combine the liquid. Cook the liver: Cook the liver for about 5 minutes, stirring occasionally, until it is well cooked and has taken on a pink color inside. Add the butter and parsley: Once cooked, add the butter in flakes and the chopped parsley. Stir gently to melt the butter and flavor the liver. Serve: Serve the Venetian liver piping hot with a side of grilled polenta or baked potatoes.

Nutritional values (per serving):

Calories: 450 kcal

Fat: 30 g

Protein: 35 g

Carbohydrates: 10 g

Fibers: 2 g

CHICKEN CURRY WITH SPINACH

Preparation time: 20 minutes

Cooking times: 25 minutes

Doses for 4 people

Ingredients:

4 chicken breasts

(from 180 g. each)

Fresh spinach (400 g)

Coconut milk (400 ml)

Curry powder (2 tablespoons)

Extra virgin olive oil (60 ml)

Salt and black pepper

Preparation:

1. Cook the chicken in a pan with olive oil until golden and cooked through. 2. Add fresh spinach and cook until wilted. 3. Pour in the coconut milk and curry powder. Cook until the chicken is cooked through and the sauce is thick. 4. Complete with salt and pepper. 5. Serve as a main course full of flavour.

Nutritional values (per serving):

Calories: 600 kcal

Fat: 30 g

Protein: 40 g

Carbohydrates: 50 g

Fibres: 5 g

BAKED SALMON WITH VEGETABLES

Preparation time: 10 minutes

Cooking time: 20 minutes

Doses: 1 person

Ingredients:

200 g of salmon fillet

100 g of potatoes

50 g of courgettes

50 g of carrots

1 red onion

1 clove of garlic

2 tablespoons extra virgin olive oil

1 tablespoon fresh herbs

chopped (rosemary, thyme, marjoram)

Salt to taste Freshly ground black pepper to taste

Preparation:

Preheat the oven to 200°C. Wash and clean the vegetables: Peel the potatoes and cut them into cubes. Wash the courgettes and cut them into rounds. Peel the carrots and cut them into rounds. Slice the red onion and mince the garlic. Season the vegetables: In a large bowl, pour the potatoes, courgettes, carrots, sliced onion and chopped garlic. Add 2 tablespoons of extra virgin olive oil, the chopped aromatic herbs, salt and pepper. Mix well to distribute the seasoning evenly. Arrange the vegetables on a baking tray. Spread the seasoned vegetables on the bottom of the pan. Prepare the salmon: Wash the salmon fillet and dry it with kitchen paper. Place it on top of the vegetables in the pan. Season the salmon with a drizzle of extra virgin olive oil, salt and pepper.

Bake: Bake the pan with the salmon and vegetables for about 20 minutes, or until the salmon is cooked and the vegetables are golden brown. Serve: Remove the baked salmon from the oven with vegetables and serve hot. If desired, it can be accompanied with a side dish of rice or quinoa.

Nutritional values (per serving):

Calories: 500 kcal

Fat: 25 g

Protein: 30 g

Carbohydrates: 40 g

Fibres: 5 g

CHICKEN WITH LEMON

Preparation time: 15 minutes

Cooking time: 10 minutes

Doses: 1 person

Ingredients:

200 g chicken breast cut into slices

1/2 untreated lemon

1 tablespoon of flour

1 tablespoon extra virgin olive oil

1/2 clove of garlic

1 sprig of rosemary, Salt to taste

Freshly ground black pepper to taste

Preparation:

Flour the chicken slices: Place the flour on a flat plate and carefully flour the chicken slices on both sides, removing any excess flour. Heat the oil in a pan:

In a large skillet, heat the extra virgin olive oil over medium-high heat. Cook the chicken: Place the floured chicken slices in the pan with the hot oil and cook them for about 2-3 minutes per side, or until golden brown. Deglaze with white wine (optional): If desired, deglaze the chicken with dry white wine. Pour the wine into the pan and stir gently to evaporate the alcohol. Add the aromas: Combine the chopped garlic, the rosemary sprig and the grated zest of 1/2 lemon. Salt and pepper to taste. Cook with lemon: Squeeze the juice of 1/2 lemon over the chicken and cook for another minute, stirring gently to combine the juice with the seasoning. Serve: Plate the lemon chicken and serve hot. Nutritional values (per portion): Calories: 300 kcal Fat: 15 g Protein: 30 g Carbohydrates: 2 g Fibre: 0.5 g

GRILLED STEAK

Preparation time: 10 minutes

Cooking time: 4-5 minutes

Doses: 1 person

Ingredients:

1 beef steak (recommended cuts:

entrecôte, sirloin,)

about 2 cm thick, Salt to taste

Freshly ground black pepper to taste

Extra virgin olive oil (optional)

Preparation:

Choosing the steak: For a perfect grilled steak, it is important to use high-quality beef. The recommended cuts are entrecôte, sirloin with a thickness of at least 2 cm. Pat the steak with kitchen paper to dry it well on both sides. Season the steak: Season with salt and

pepper steak generously on both sides. Cook the steak: Place the steak on the hot grill and cook for 2-3 minutes per side for medium rare (rare). For more or less toasted cooking, adjust the cooking time according to your tastes. Turn the steak only once: If desired, brush the steak with a drizzle of extra virgin olive oil during cooking to make it shinier and tastier. Resting time: Once cooked, remove the steak from the grill and let it rest for 2-3 minutes on a cutting board before serving. This will allow the juices to distribute evenly throughout the meat. Nutritional values (per serving):

Calories: 350 kcal

Fat: 20 g

Protein: 30 g

Carbohydrates: 0 g

TURKEY BURGER

Preparation time: 20 minutes

Cooking time: 15 minutes

Servings: 2 burgers

Ingredients:

300 g of minced turkey

1 tablespoon breadcrumbs

1 egg

1 small white onion chopped

1 clove of minced garlic

1 tablespoon chopped fresh parsley

1/2 teaspoon dried oregano

1/4 teaspoon cumin powder

Salt to taste

Freshly ground black pepper to taste

4 tablespoons of extra virgin olive oil

Preparation:

Prepare the hamburger mixture: In a large bowl mix the ground turkey, breadcrumbs, egg, chopped onion, chopped garlic, chopped parsley, dried oregano, ground cumin, salt and pepper. Mix the mixture well with your hands until you obtain a smooth mixture. Form the burgers: Divide the mixture into 4 equal portions and use your hands to form 4 burgers of approximately 10 cm in diameter and 2 cm thick. If the mixture is too sticky, moisten your hands slightly. Cook the burgers: Heat the extra virgin olive oil in a nonstick skillet over medium-high heat. Cook the burgers for about 3-4 minutes per side, or until browned and cooked through.

Assemble the burgers: Toast the hamburger buns. Fill the buns with the cooked burgers, sliced tomato, green lettuce, sliced red onion, cheddar, ketchup, mayonnaise and mustard (to taste). Serve: Serve the turkey burgers piping hot.

Nutritional values (per hamburger):

Calories: 350 kcal

Fat: 20 g

Protein: 30 g

Carbohydrates: 10 g

GRILLED CHICKEN BREAST

Preparation time: 15 minutes

Cooking time: 10 minutes

Doses: 1 person

Ingredients:

150 g of chicken breast

1/2 tablespoon extra virgin olive oil

Salt to taste

Freshly ground black pepper to taste

Preparation:

Prepare the chicken breast: Rinse the chicken breast under running water and dry it with kitchen paper. Remove any cuticles or excess fat. Season the chicken breast: In a large bowl, pour the chicken breast, extra virgin olive oil, a pinch of salt and a grind of black pepper.

Mix well to make the seasoning adhere to the entire surface of the chicken. Cook the chicken breast: Heat a grill over medium-high heat. Place the chicken breast on the hot grill and cook for about 4-5 minutes per side, or until golden brown and cooked through. It is important not to pierce the chicken with a fork during cooking to prevent it from losing its juices. Serve:

Nutritional values (per serving):

Calories: 250 kcal

Fat: 10 g

Protein: 35 g

Carbohydrates: 0 g

BAKED TROUT

Preparation time: 20 minutes

Cooking time: 20 minutes

Doses: 1 person

Ingredients:

1 salmon trout weighing approximately 250 g

2 tablespoons extra virgin olive oil

1 untreated lemon

1 clove of garlic

1 sprig of rosemary

1/2 teaspoon dried oregano

Salt to taste

Freshly ground black pepper to taste

Cherry tomatoes (optional)

Black olives (optional)

Preparation:

Clean the trout: Wash the trout carefully under running water and dry it with kitchen paper. Remove the scales if present, gut it and wash it inside again. Season the trout: In a large bowl pour the extra virgin olive oil, the juice of a lemon, the chopped garlic, the chopped rosemary, the dried oregano, a pinch of salt and a grind of black pepper. Mix the seasoning well. Arrange the trout on a baking tray: Place the trout on a baking tray lined with baking paper. Distribute the seasoning inside the abdominal cavity and on the surface of the trout.

Bake: Preheat the oven to 180°C. Cook the trout in a static oven for about 20 minutes, or until the skin is golden brown and the meat is completely cooked. Serve: Remove the baked trout from the oven and serve hot.

Nutritional values (per serving):

Calories: 350 kcal

Fat: 20 g

Protein: 30 g

Carbohydrates: 5 g

VEGETABLE OMELETTE

Preparation time: 10 minutes

Cooking time: 15 minutes

Doses: 1 person

Ingredients:

2 eggs

1 tablespoon grated parmesan

1/4 white onion chopped

50 g of mixed vegetables of your choice (courgettes,

peppers, aubergines, tomatoes, etc.)

1 tablespoon extra virgin olive oil

Salt to taste

Freshly ground black pepper to taste

Chopped fresh chives (optional)

Preparation:

Beat the eggs: In a large bowl, beat the eggs with a pinch of salt and pepper. Add the parmesan: Combine the grated parmesan with the beaten eggs and mix well. Prepare the vegetables: Wash and cut the chosen vegetables into small pieces. In a non-stick pan, heat the extra virgin olive oil and fry the chopped onion for a couple of minutes. Add the mixed vegetables and cook for about 5-10 minutes, or until softened. Make the omelette: Pour the beaten egg mixture into the pan with the cooked vegetables. Distribute the vegetables evenly in the batter. Cook the omelette: Cook the omelette over low heat for about 7-8 minutes, or until the edges begin to pull away from the pan.

Turn and complete cooking: Using a plate or lid, turn the omelette and cook it for another minute to brown it on the other side too. **Serve:** Fold the omelette in half or into a triangle and serve hot, garnished with chopped fresh chives (optional).

Nutritional values (per serving):

Calories: 250 kcal

Fat: 15 g

Protein: 15 g

Carbohydrates: 5 g

GRILLED SHRIMP AND VEGETABLES SKEWERS

Preparation time: 20 minutes

Cooking time: 15 minutes

Doses for 2 people

Ingredients:

12 shrimp

1 courgette

1 red pepper

1 red onion

2 tablespoons of oil

extra virgin olive oil

Salt and Pepper To Taste

Preparation:

Clean the prawns and shell them, leaving the tail intact. Wash the vegetables and cut them into cubes of about 2 cm. In a bowl, mix the extra virgin olive oil with salt and pepper. Marinate the shrimp and vegetables in the bowl for 15 minutes. Thread the prawns and vegetables onto the skewers alternating them. Cook the skewers on a hot grill for 5 minutes per side, or until the prawns are fully cooked. Serve the skewers hot. Nutritional values (per serving):

Calories: 300

Fat: 15 g

Protein: 30 g

Carbohydrates: 10 g

CHICKEN THIGHS WITH CURRY WITH GREEK YOGURT

Preparation time: 20 minutes

Cooking time: 30 minutes

Doses for 2 people

Ingredients:

2 chicken thighs

1 tablespoon curry powder

1 white onion

1 clove of garlic

200 g of Greek yogurt

1 tablespoon of oil

extra virgin olive oil

Salt and Pepper To Taste

Preparation:

In a bowl, mix the curry powder with salt and pepper. Rub the curry mixture over the chicken thighs. In a non-stick pan, heat the extra virgin olive oil and fry the chopped onion and chopped garlic for 5 minutes. Add the chicken thighs and cook for 10 minutes per side. Add the Greek yogurt and cook for another 10 minutes, stirring occasionally. Serve the chicken legs with the curry gravy. Nutritional values (per serving):

Calories: 400

Fat: 20 g

Protein: 40 g

Carbohydrates: 10 g

SEABASS IN PAPER WITH OLIVES AND TOMATOES

Preparation time: 20 minutes

Cooking time: 20 minutes

Doses for 2 people

Ingredients:

2 sea bass fillets

100 g of cherry tomatoes

50 g of black olives

1 sprig of thyme

1 tablespoon of oil

extra virgin olive oil

Salt and Pepper To Taste

Preparation:

Preheat the oven to 180°C. Wash the cherry tomatoes and cut them in half. Rinse the olives and pit them. Arrange the sea bass fillets on a sheet of baking paper. Distribute the cherry tomatoes, olives and thyme over the sea bass fillets. Season with extra virgin olive oil, salt and pepper. Close the package and seal it well. Bake in the oven for 20 minutes. Serve the sea bass hot in foil.

Nutritional values (per serving):

Calories: 350

Fat: 15 g

Protein: 35 g

Carbohydrates: 10 g

GRILLED TUNA SLICE WITH AVOCADO SAUCE

Preparation time: 20 minutes

Cooking time: 15 minutes

Doses for 2 people

Ingredients:

2 tuna steaks, 150 g each

1 avocado

1 lime

1/2 red onion

1 jalapeño pepper

1 tablespoon chopped coriander

Extra virgin olive oil

Salt and Pepper To Taste

Preparation:

Preheat grill to medium-high heat. Season the tuna steaks with extra virgin olive oil, salt and pepper. Cook the tuna steaks on the grill for 5 minutes per side, or until desired doneness. In a bowl, mash the avocado with a fork. Add the lime juice, finely chopped red onion, finely chopped jalapeño pepper and chopped cilantro. Mix well and season with salt and pepper. Serve the tuna steak with the avocado sauce.

Nutritional values (per serving):

Calories: 400

Fat: 30 g

Protein: 40 g

SALMON IN ALMOND CRUST

Preparation time: 20 minutes

Cooking time: 15 minutes

Doses for 2 people

Ingredients:

2 salmon steaks (200 g each)

50 g of flaked almonds

1 egg white

1 tablespoon of oil

extra virgin olive oil

Salt and Pepper To Taste

Preparation:

Preheat the oven to 200°C Brush the salmon steaks with egg white. Sprinkle the salmon steaks with the flaked almonds, pressing lightly to make them adhere. Season with salt and pepper. Arrange the salmon steaks on a baking tray lined with baking paper. Drizzle with a drizzle of extra virgin olive oil. Bake for 15 minutes, or until salmon is fully cooked. Serve the almond crusted salmon hot. Nutritional values (per serving):

Calories: 400

Fat: 25 g

Protein: 30 g

Carbohydrates: 5 g

CHICKEN BREAST STUFFED WITH ARTICHOKES

Preparation time: 30 minutes

Cooking time: 40 minutes

Doses for 2 people

Ingredients:

2 chicken breasts

2 artichokes

1 shallot

1 clove of garlic

1 tablespoon chopped parsley

50 g of breadcrumbs

50 g of grated Grana Padano

2 tablespoons extra virgin olive oil

Salt and Pepper To Taste

Preparation:

Clean the artichokes and cut them into thin slices. Fry the chopped shallot and chopped garlic in a pan with extra virgin olive oil over medium heat. Add the artichokes and cook for 10 minutes. Salt and pepper to taste. Cut the chicken breasts into pockets and stuff them with the artichoke mixture. Close the pockets with toothpicks. In a bowl, mix the breadcrumbs with the grated Grana Padano, the chopped parsley, salt and pepper. Bread the chicken breasts in the breadcrumb mixture. Arrange the chicken breasts on a baking tray. Drizzle with a drizzle of extra virgin olive oil. Bake at 180°C for 40 minutes, or until the chicken is fully cooked. Serve the chicken breast stuffed with hot artichokes. Nutritional values (per serving): Calories: 500. Fat: 30 g

Proteins: 40 g, Carbohydrates: 10 g

AUBERGINES ROLLS

Preparation time: 30 minutes

Cooking time: 40 minutes

Doses: 1 person

Ingredients:

1 medium aubergine

1/2 tablespoon extra virgin olive oil

Salt to taste

Freshly ground black pepper to taste

50 g of ricotta

20 g of grated mozzarella

1 tablespoon chopped fresh basil

200 g of tomato puree

1 clove of garlic

1 tablespoon extra virgin olive oil

Preparation:

Prepare the aubergines: Wash the aubergine and cut it into thin longitudinal slices about 1/2 cm thick. Arrange the aubergine slices on a baking tray lined with baking paper, brush them with a drizzle of extra virgin olive oil, lightly salt and pepper them. Cook in a preheated fan oven at 180°C for about 20 minutes, or until the aubergines are softened and lightly golden. Prepare the filling: In a bowl mix the ricotta with the grated mozzarella, chopped basil, a pinch of salt and ground black pepper. Mix the mixture well until you obtain a homogeneous mixture. Assemble the rolls: Take a slice of cooked aubergine and spread a spoonful of filling on one side. Roll the aubergine slice on itself to form a roll. Proceed in the same way for all the aubergine slices. Prepare the sauce: In a pan, heat the extra virgin olive oil and fry the minced garlic for a minute. Add the tomato puree, a pinch of salt and a grind of black pepper. Cook over low heat for about 15 minutes, stirring occasionally. Cook the rolls: Pour a spoonful of tomato sauce on the bottom of a baking tray. Arrange the aubergine rolls in the pan and pour the remaining sauce over them. Cook in a preheated static oven at 180°C for about 15 minutes, or until the sauce is thickened and the rolls are hot. Serve: Remove the aubergine rolls from the oven and serve them piping hot, accompanied by a side dish of fresh vegetables or bread.

Nutritional values (per serving):

Calories: 350 kcal

Fat: 20 g

Protein: 20 g

Carbohydrates: 30 g

BAKED CHICKEN WITH TOMATOES AND OLIVES

Preparation time: 20 minutes

Cooking time: 40 minutes

Doses for 2 people

Ingredients:

2 chicken thighs

200 g of cherry tomatoes

100 g of black olives

1 sprig of rosemary

1 tablespoon of oil

extra virgin olive oil

Salt and Pepper To Taste

Preparation:

Preheat the oven to 180°C. Place the chicken legs on a baking tray. Add the cherry tomatoes cut in half, the black olives and the rosemary. Season with extra virgin olive oil, salt and pepper. Bake for 40 minutes, or until chicken is fully cooked. Serve the baked chicken with hot cherry tomatoes and olives. Nutritional values (per serving):

Calories: 400

Fat: 25 g

Protein: 30 g

Carbohydrates: 10 g

BAKED COD WITH OLIVES
AND TOMATOES

Preparation time: 20 minutes

Cooking time: 20 minutes

Doses for 2 people

Ingredients:

2 cod fillets (200 g each)

100 g of cherry tomatoes

50 g of black olives

1 sprig of rosemary

1 tablespoon of oil

extra virgin olive oil

Salt and Pepper To Taste

Preparation:

Preheat the oven to 180°C. Arrange the cod fillets on a baking tray. Add the cherry tomatoes cut in half, the black olives and the rosemary. Season with extra virgin olive oil, salt and pepper. Bake for 20 minutes, or until the cod is fully cooked. Serve the baked cod with olives and hot cherry tomatoes. If you prefer, you can also cook the cod in the oven with the potatoes. In this case, add the diced potatoes to the pan together with the cod and cook for about 30 minutes. Nutritional values (per serving):

Calories: 350

Fat: 20 g

Protein: 30 g

Carbohydrates: 10 g

RECIPES SIDE DISH

SPINACH AND ALMOND SALAD

Preparation time: 10 minutes

Cooking time: 0 minutes

Doses for 2 people:

Ingredients

200 g of fresh spinach

50 g of shelled almonds

20 g of grated parmesan

1 tablespoon extra virgin olive oil

Lemon juice (optional)

Salt to taste

Freshly ground black pepper to taste

Preparation:

Wash the spinach well and dry them with a cloth. Toast the almonds in a non-stick pan for a couple of minutes, stirring often, until golden. In a large bowl, combine the spinach, toasted almonds, grated parmesan, extra virgin olive oil, lemon juice (if using), a pinch of salt and ground black pepper. Mix everything well and serve the salad immediately.

Nutritional values (per serving):

Calories: 300 kcal

Fat: 20 g

Protein: 15 g

Carbohydrates: 10 g

GRILLED COURGETTES WITH LEMON AND MINT

Preparation time: 15 minutes

Cooking time: 10 minutes

Doses for 2 people:

Ingredients

2 medium courgettes

1 tablespoon extra virgin olive oil

Lemon juice (optional)

Salt to taste

Freshly ground black pepper to taste

Fresh mint leaves (optional)

Preparation:

Wash the courgettes and cut them into thin slices. Heat a grill or non-stick pan. Lightly grease the grill or pan with extra virgin olive oil. Cook grilled courgettes for 5 minutes per side, or until golden brown. Season the grilled courgettes with a drizzle of extra virgin olive oil, lemon juice (if using), a pinch of salt and freshly ground black pepper. Decorate with fresh mint leaves (optional) and serve immediately.

Nutritional values (per serving):

Calories: 150 kcal

Fat: 10 g

Protein: 2 g

Carbohydrates: 5 g

TOMATOES STUFFED WITH COUSCOUS

Preparation time: 20 minutes

Cooking time: 20 minutes

Doses for 2 people:

Ingredients:

4 medium tomatoes

100 g of couscous

150 ml of vegetable broth

1/2 red onion

1 green pepper

1 small courgette

1 tablespoon extra virgin olive oil

Fresh basil

Salt to taste

Freshly ground black pepper to taste

Preparation:

Wash the tomatoes and cut them in half horizontally, removing the seeds and internal pulp. Prepare the couscous: pour the couscous into a large bowl, add a pinch of salt and fluff with the tines of a fork. Pour the hot vegetable broth over the couscous, mix well and cover with a cloth. Leave to rest for 10 minutes. Finely chop the red onion. Cut the green pepper and courgette into small pieces. In a pan, heat the extra virgin olive oil and fry the chopped onion for a couple of minutes. Add the green pepper and courgette and cook for about 5 minutes, or until the vegetables are softened. Fluff the couscous with a fork and add it to the vegetables in the pan. Mix well and cook for a couple of minutes, stirring often.

Add the chopped fresh basil leaves, a pinch of salt and ground black pepper to the couscous mixture. Fill the tomatoes with the couscous and vegetable mixture. Arrange the stuffed tomatoes on a baking tray greased with extra virgin olive oil. Cook in a preheated static oven at 180°C for about 20 minutes, or until the tomatoes are golden brown. Serve the tomatoes stuffed with couscous piping hot.

Nutritional values (per serving):

Calories: 350 kcal

Fat: 15 g

Protein: 15 g

Carbohydrates: 35 g

ICE CARROTS WITH HONEY

Preparation time: 10 minutes

Cooking time: 20 minutes

Doses for 2 people:

Ingredients:

4 medium carrots

2 tablespoons honey

1 tablespoon butter

1/2 teaspoon ground cinnamon

Salt to taste

Freshly ground black pepper to taste

Preparation:

Wash the carrots and peel them. Cut the carrots into rounds about 1 cm thick. In a pan, heat the butter over medium heat. Add the carrots and cook them for about 5 minutes, stirring often. Combine the honey, ground cinnamon, a pinch of salt and ground black pepper. Mix well and cook for a further 15 minutes, or until the carrots are tender and caramelised. Serve the honey-glazed carrots piping hot.

Nutritional values (per serving):

Calories: 200 kcal

Fat: 10 g

Protein: 1 g

Carbohydrates: 30 g

SPINACH SALAD WITH TOMATOES AND FETA

Preparation time: 10 minutes

Cooking time: 0 minutes

Doses for 2 people

Ingredients:

200 g of fresh spinach

150 g of cherry tomatoes

100 g of feta

1 red onion

3 tablespoons of oil

extra virgin olive oil

1 tablespoon lemon juice

Salt and Pepper To Taste

Preparation:

Wash the spinach and dry them well. Cut the cherry tomatoes in half. Crumble the feta. Slice the red onion. In a bowl, mix the spinach, cherry tomatoes, feta, red onion, extra virgin olive oil, lemon juice, salt and pepper. Serve the spinach salad with cherry tomatoes and feta immediately.

Nutritional values (per serving):

Calories: 200

Fat: 15 g

Protein: 15 g

Carbohydrates: 10 g

BAKED BROCCOLI WITH PARMESAN

Preparation time: 20 minutes

Cooking time: 20 minutes

Doses for 2 people

Ingredients:

500 g of broccoli

50 g of grated parmesan

2 tablespoons of oil

extra virgin olive oil

Salt and Pepper To Taste

Preparation:

Preheat the oven to 200°C. Wash the broccoli and cut them into florets. Arrange the broccoli on a baking tray. Season with extra virgin olive oil, salt and pepper. Sprinkle the broccoli with the grated parmesan. Bake for 20 minutes, or until broccoli is golden brown. Nutritional values (per serving):

Calories: 250

Fat: 15 g

Protein: 20 g

Carbohydrates: 15 g

PAN-FRIED BRUSSELS SPROUTS

Preparation time: 15 minutes

Cooking time: 10 minutes

Doses for 2 people:

Ingredients:

300 g of Brussels sprouts

1 tablespoon extra virgin olive oil

1 clove of garlic

1/2 hot pepper (optional)

Salt to taste

Freshly ground

black pepper to taste

Preparation:

Wash the Brussels sprouts and cut them in half. In a pan, heat the extra virgin olive oil over medium heat. Add the minced garlic and hot pepper (if using) and fry for a minute. Add the Brussels sprouts and cook them for about 5 minutes, stirring often. Salt and pepper to taste. Cook for an additional 5 minutes, or until the Brussels sprouts are tender. Serve the pan-fried Brussels sprouts piping hot.

Nutritional values (per serving):

Calories: 150 kcal

Fat: 10 g

Protein: 5 g

Carbohydrates: 10 g

ROASTED PEPPERS WITH GARLIC

Preparation time: 15 minutes

Cooking time: 40 minutes

Doses for 2 people:

Ingredients:

2 peppers

2 tablespoons extra virgin olive oil

2 cloves of garlic

Salt to taste

Freshly ground black pepper to taste

Preparation:

Wash the peppers and cut them in half lengthwise, removing the seeds and white filaments. Arrange the peppers on a baking tray lined with baking paper. Drizzle the peppers with a drizzle of oil

extra virgin olive oil. Add the peeled and lightly crushed garlic cloves. Salt and pepper to taste. Cook in a preheated static oven at 180°C for about 40 minutes, or until the peppers are well roasted and soft. Remove the roasted peppers from the oven and let them cool slightly. Peel the roasted peppers (optional). Cut the roasted peppers into strips.

Serve the roasted peppers with garlic hot.

Nutritional values (per serving):

Calories: 100 kcal

Fat: 5 g

Protein: 2 g

Carbohydrates: 15 g

PAN-FRIED GREEN BEANS
WITH SHALLOTS

Preparation time: 15 minutes

Cooking time: 15 minutes

Doses for 2 people

Ingredients:

300 g of green beans

1 shallot

2 tablespoons of oil

extra virgin olive oil

Salt and Pepper To Taste

Preparation:

Wash the green beans and trim them. Cook the green beans in boiling salted water for 10 minutes. Remove the green beans and cool them under running water. Cut the shallot into thin slices. Heat the extra virgin olive oil in a pan over medium heat. Fry the shallot for 2 minutes. Add the green beans and cook for 5 minutes, stirring frequently. Salt and pepper to taste. Serve the pan-fried green beans with shallots hot.

Nutritional values (per serving):

Calories: 150

Fat: 10 g

Protein: 10 g

Carbohydrates: 10 g

GRILLED MARINATED COURGETTES

Preparation time: 20 minutes

Cooking time: 15 minutes

Doses for 2 people

Ingredients:

2 courgettes

2 tablespoons of oil

extra virgin olive oil

1 tablespoon lemon juice

1 clove of garlic

1 sprig of thyme

Salt and Pepper To Taste

Preparation:

Wash the courgettes and cut them into slices. Heat a grill over medium-high heat. Grill the courgettes for 5 minutes per side, or until golden brown. In a bowl, mix the extra virgin olive oil, lemon juice, chopped garlic, chopped thyme, salt and pepper. Marinate the grilled courgettes in the sauce for 15 minutes. Serve the marinated grilled courgettes.

Nutritional values (per serving):

Calories: 100

Fat: 5 g

Protein: 5 g

Carbohydrates: 5 g

SAUTEED MUSHROOMS WITH PARSLEY

Preparation time: 15 minutes

Cooking time: 10 minutes

Doses for 2 people:

Ingredients:

300 g of mixed mushrooms

1 tablespoon extra virgin olive oil

1 clove of garlic

1/2 shallot

1/2 glass of dry white wine (optional)

Fresh parsley

Salt to taste

Freshly ground black pepper to taste

Preparation:

Clean the mushrooms and cut them into slices. In a pan, heat the extra virgin olive oil over medium heat. Add the chopped garlic and finely chopped shallots and fry for a minute. Add the mushrooms and cook them for about 5 minutes, stirring often. Add the dry white wine (if used) and let it evaporate. Salt and pepper to taste. Cook for an additional 5 minutes, or until the mushrooms are tender. Add the chopped fresh parsley and mix well. Serve the sautéed mushrooms with parsley hot.

Nutritional values (per serving):

Calories: 150 kcal

Fat: 10 g

Protein: 5 g

Carbohydrates: 10 g

STEAMED ASPARAGUS WITH PARMESAN

Preparation time: 10 minutes

Cooking time: 10 minutes

Doses for 2 people:

Ingredients:

200 g of asparagus

Waterfall

Grated Parmesan cheese

Salt to taste

Freshly ground black pepper to taste

Preparation:

Wash the asparagus and cut the hard end part. Steam the asparagus for 10 minutes, or until tender. Arrange the cooked asparagus on a serving platter. Drizzle the asparagus with a drizzle of extra virgin olive oil. Sprinkle with grated parmesan to taste. Salt and pepper to taste. Serve the steamed asparagus with parmesan piping hot.

Nutritional values (per serving):

Calories: 100 kcal

Fat: 5 g

Protein: 5 g

Carbohydrates: 10 g

ROASTED CAULIFLOWER WITH CURRY

Preparation time: 20 minutes

Cooking time: 30 minutes

Doses for 2 people

Ingredients:

1 cauliflower

2 tablespoons curry powder

2 tablespoons of oil

extra virgin olive oil

Salt and Pepper To Taste

Preparation:

Preheat the oven to 200°C. Cut the cauliflower into florets. In a bowl, mix the curry, extra virgin olive oil, salt and pepper. Add the cauliflower florets to the bowl and mix well. Arrange the cauliflower florets on a baking tray. Bake for 30 minutes, or until the cauliflower is golden and crisp.

Nutritional values (per serving):

Calories: 200

Fat: 10 g

Protein: 10 g

Carbohydrates: 20 g

BAKED CARROTS WITH HONEY AND ROSEMARY

Preparation time: 15 minutes

Cooking time: 20 minutes

Doses for 2 people

Ingredients:

500 g of carrots

2 tablespoons honey

1 sprig of rosemary

Salt and Pepper To Taste

Preparation:

Preheat the oven to 200°C. Peel the carrots and cut them into rounds. In a bowl, mix the honey, chopped rosemary, salt and pepper. Add the carrot slices to the bowl and mix well. Arrange the carrot rounds on a baking tray. Bake for 20 minutes, or until carrots are soft.

Nutritional values (per serving):

Calories: 150

Fat: 5 g

Protein: 5 g

Carbohydrates: 25 g

BAKED BEET WITH YOGURT SAUCE

Preparation time: 20 minutes

Cooking time: 45 minutes

Doses for 2 people

Ingredients:

2 beets

100 g of Greek yogurt

1 tablespoon of oil

extra virgin olive oil

1 clove of garlic

1 sprig of mint

Salt and Pepper To Taste

Preparation:

Preheat the oven to 200°C. Wash the beets and wrap them individually in foil. Bake the beets in the oven for 45 minutes, or until soft. In a bowl, mix the Greek yogurt, extra virgin olive oil, chopped garlic, chopped mint, salt and pepper. Remove the beets from the oven and peel them. Cut the beets into slices and serve with the yogurt sauce.

Nutritional values (per serving):

Calories: 250

Fat: 10 g

Protein: 15 g

Carbohydrates: 30 g

BAKED SWEET POTATOES WITH PAPRIKA

Preparation time: 15 minutes

Cooking time: 30 minutes

Doses for 2 people

Ingredients:

2 sweet potatoes

1 tablespoon paprika

1 tablespoon of oil

extra virgin olive oil

Salt and Pepper To Taste

Preparation:

Preheat the oven to 200°C. Peel the sweet potatoes and cut them into cubes. In a bowl, mix the paprika, extra virgin olive oil, salt and pepper. Add the sweet potato cubes to the bowl and mix well. Arrange the sweet potato cubes on a baking sheet. Bake for 30 minutes, or until the sweet potatoes are golden brown and crisp.

Nutritional values (per serving):

Calories: 200

Fat: 10 g

Protein: 5 g

Carbohydrates: 30 g

BAKED PUMPKIN WITH SAGE AND WALNUTS

Preparation time: 20 minutes

Cooking time: 40 minutes

Doses for 4 people

Ingredients:

1 kg of pumpkin

10 sage leaves

50 g of walnuts

4 tablespoons of oil

extra virgin olive oil

Salt and Pepper To Taste

Preparation:

Preheat the oven to 200°C. Wash the pumpkin and cut it into slices about 2 cm thick. Arrange the pumpkin slices on a baking tray. Spread the sage leaves and walnuts over the pumpkin slices. Season with extra virgin olive oil, salt and pepper. Bake for 40 minutes, or until squash is soft.

Nutritional values (per serving):

Calories: 250

Fat: 15 g

Protein: 5 g

Carbohydrates: 30 g

QUINOA SALAD WITH VEGETABLES AND FETA

Preparation time: 20 minutes

Cooking time: 20 minutes

Doses for 4 people

Ingredients:

200 g of quinoa

200 g of cherry tomatoes

1 cucumber

1 red pepper

1 red onion

150 g of feta

4 tablespoons of extra virgin olive oil

2 tablespoons lemon juice

Salt and Pepper To Taste

Preparation:

Cook the quinoa in boiling salted water for 20 minutes. Drain the quinoa and cool it under running water. Cut the cherry tomatoes in half. Cut the cucumber into cubes. Cut the red pepper into cubes. Cut the red onion into thin slices. Crumble the feta. In a bowl, mix the quinoa, cherry tomatoes, cucumber, red bell pepper, red onion, feta, extra virgin olive oil, lemon juice, salt and pepper.

Nutritional values (per serving):

Calories: 400

Fat: 20 g

Protein: 20 g

Carbohydrates: 40 g

CUCUMBER AND AVOCADO SALAD

Preparation time: 10 minutes

Cooking time: 0 minutes

Doses for 2 people:

Ingredients:

1 medium cucumber

1 ripe avocado

1/2 red onion

1 tomato

1 tablespoon extra virgin olive oil

Lemon juice (optional)

Salt to taste

Freshly ground black pepper to taste

Preparation:

Wash the cucumber and cut it into thin slices. Cut the avocado in half, remove the stone and peel and cut the pulp into cubes. Cut the red onion into thin slices. Cut the tomato into small pieces. In a large bowl, combine the cucumber, avocado, red onion, tomato, extra virgin olive oil, lemon juice (if using), a pinch of salt and freshly ground black pepper. Mix everything well and serve the cucumber and avocado salad immediately.

Nutritional values (per serving):

Calories: 250 kcal

Fat: 20 g

Protein: 5 g

Carbohydrates: 15 g

GRILLED AUBERGINES WITH BASIL

Preparation time: 20 minutes

Cooking time: 20 minutes

Doses for 2 people:

Ingredients:

2 medium aubergines

2 tablespoons extra virgin olive oil

Fresh basil

Salt to taste

Freshly ground black pepper to taste

Preparation:

Wash the aubergines and cut them into slices about 1 cm thick. Sprinkle the aubergine slices with a pinch of salt. In a pan, heat the extra virgin olive oil over medium heat. Cook the grilled aubergines for about 10 minutes per side, or until golden brown. Arrange the grilled aubergines on a serving plate. Drizzle the grilled aubergines with a drizzle of extra virgin olive oil. Decorate with fresh basil leaves. Salt and pepper to taste. Serve the grilled aubergines with basil piping hot.

Nutritional values (per serving):

Calories: 200 kcal

Fat: 15 g

Protein: 5 g

Carbohydrates: 10 g

CONCLUSION

Thank you for embarking on this journey with "OMAD Diet 2025". We hope the book has given you all the information, tools, and inspiration you need to transform your life through the OMAD approach. Adopting a new lifestyle may seem like a challenge, but with determination and the right resources, the benefits can be extraordinary. We explored together the fundamental principles of the OMAD diet, its many benefits, weekly meal plans, and delicious recipes to help you maintain optimal nutritional balance.

Through testimonials and practical advice, we hope to have given you the confidence needed to start and persevere on this path. Your feedback is valuable to us and to everyone who is looking for reliable information and inspiration. We kindly invite you to share your experience and opinions by leaving a review.

Your words can make a difference to other readers who are considering adopting the OMAD diet.

Note: We would be grateful if you could take a few minutes to leave a review. Your opinions help us to improve and always offer the best to our readers. Thank you again for choosing "OMAD Diet 2025". We wish you health, happiness and success on your journey to a better future. We can't wait to hear your opinion! With gratitude,

[KLARLOCK]

9 798332 725913